Promoting Successful Aging

AAW 1950

Lucinda Lee Roff
Charles R. Atherton

University of Alabama

D0862180

Nelson-Hall Series in Social Welfare

Consulting editor: **Charles Zastrow**
University of Wisconsin-Whitewater

Nelson-Hall **nh** Chicago

Project Editor: Dorothy Anderson
Copy Editor: Elizabeth Rubenstein
Designer: Claudia von Hendricks
Cover Design: Richard Meade, Claudia von Hendricks
Photo Research: Stephen Forsling
Manufacturer: Braun-Brumfield, Inc.
Cover Painting: *Cotton Candy Days*
by Audrey Langer

LIBRARY OF CONGRESS CATALOGING-IN-PUBLICATION DATA

Roff, Lucinda Lee.
    Promoting successful aging / Lucinda Lee Roff, Charles R.
Atherton
        p.   cm.
    Bibliography: p.
    Includes index.
    ISBN 0-8304-1167-4
    1. Aged—Services for—United States.   2. Aged—Care—United
States.   3. Aged—United States—Social conditions.   4. Aged—Health
and hygiene—United States.   I. Atherton, Charles R.   II. Title.
HV1461.R63   1989
362.6'0973—dc19   88-38387
                                                                      CIP

Manufactured in the United States of America

10   9   8   7   6   5   4   3   2

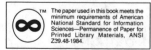

Contents

causes the older person to move toward a realistic and satisfying goal? • The Bensons • The Phillips family • Mr. Hayes

Introduction

This book is about services to older people. It is intended to help prepare people to work with older people in a variety of settings. We think that it will be most helpful to beginning social workers, nurses, recreation leaders, physical and occupational therapists, and educators, but it should also be useful to other professionals and to volunteers who work with the aging.

A key factor in working with older people is the attitude that the helping person brings to his or her tasks. Therefore, we have focused on the notion of successful aging. We would like you to learn to have a positive view of older people and to look for their strengths.

Although this is not a text in gerontology—the study of aging—we have tried to include enough information about older people to provide a context in which to work with them. Most of this information is contained in the first six chapters.

Chapter 1 reviews the current status of the aged in the United States. We have provided a sociodemographic profile of aging Americans and information about some important subpopulations. We have also set forth our beliefs about what we regard as the components of successful aging. These components are amplified in the following five chapters.

In chapter 2, we share our perspective on older persons. We are frankly trying to make converts to what we believe is a positive and constructive view of the older person. How one approaches a service population is important. We think that if people have negative attitudes toward the aging, service will inevitably suffer. Therefore, we want you to have a basis for viewing older people in the most positive light.

There are a number of important aspects to successful aging. In chapter 3, we look at the economic aspects of the older person's life and discuss the major private and public resources available to promote successful aging. Chapter 4 focuses on the health of older persons and discusses the major health problems that can affect a person's ability to age successfully. Chapter 5 reviews the structural barriers to satisfactory mental health and the major categories of problems that affect the mental health of older persons. In chapter 6, we look at the living environment of older persons and the ways in which it can be improved.

Chapter 7 outlines a general approach to working with older people. This approach is consumer oriented. Our accent is on helping people function in ways they choose as best for them, rather than in ways that are considered best by someone else. This general approach is extended in the following five chapters.

Chapter 8 focuses on working with individuals. Chapter 9 discusses working with families on behalf of older persons, and chapter 10 deals with working with groups. In chapters 6 through 10, we discuss the principles involved and try to show you how they work in practice through a series of fictional case vignettes that we have written for the purpose.

In order to work with individuals, families, and groups, one has to know about community resources. We identify a wide range of resources in chapter 11 and discuss how to use them and how to help develop new ones when they are needed.

For some older Americans, long-term care will be needed, either in their own homes or in institutions. The issues in long-term care are discussed in chapter 12. Included is a discussion of case management that enables some older people to remain in their own homes and a discussion of nursing home care. Again, vignettes are used to illustrate the major points.

A brief postscript offers some suggestions for extending your education in working with the aging.

We are committed to improving the way in which the aging are viewed. We are also committed to improving both the public and the voluntary services that promote successful aging. We hope that when you have finished this book that you will be too. We are all growing older; we are the aged of the future.

Promoting Successful Aging

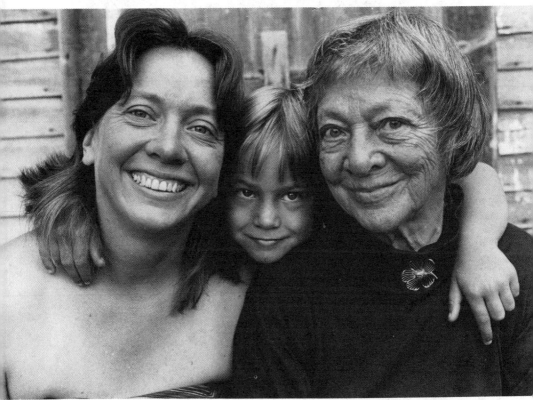

© Marianne Gontarz

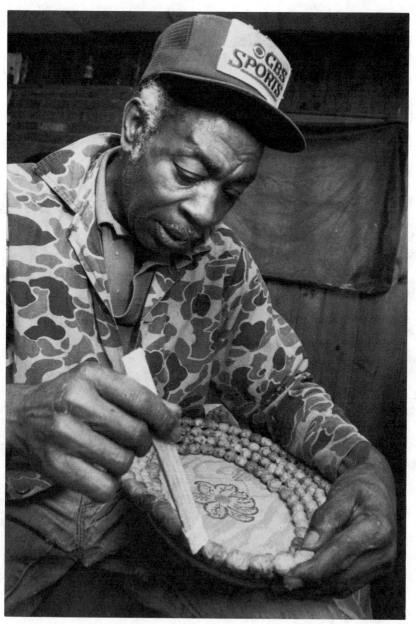

©Dan Chidester The Image Works

1

The Aged in the United States

As Act I, Scene I, of *The Tragedy of King Lear* opens, an aging Lear has gathered his three daughters in order to divide his kingdom. Shakespeare has him say:

> Know we have divided
> In three our kingdom: and 'tis our fast intent
> To shake all cares and business from our age,
> Conferring them on younger strengths, while we
> Unburthen'd crawl toward death.

While most aging persons do not have a kingdom to divide, they may well find themselves expected to act as King Lear planned to do—to shake all cares and business, get out of the way of the coming generation, and crawl quietly toward death.

This is not the view of aging that we promote in this and succeeding chapters. If we were to adopt a literary motif for our approach, we would turn to Dylan Thomas rather than Shakespeare, and urge older Americans, "Do not go gentle into that good night."

Most older Americans do not need this advice, because they are relatively well, happy, active, and involved with life. However, there are still large numbers of Americans who have difficult older years. Many of these Americans have a bad time of it not as an automatic consequence of aging, but because of unenlightened public policy. Public policy is unenlightened partly, we think, because the American public does not have the proper view of aging. While we do not pretend that we can solve the entire problem, we do think that it will help if those who work with older people have a more constructive view.

We have three central tasks in this book. First, we will present a picture of the aging as we know them. This is not an unbiased view. We clearly are on the side of the older American. And we are becoming more partisan as we grow closer to being older Americans ourselves!

Second, we will look at the state of social policy as it affects older Americans in a number of areas of life (including income, health care, and living arrangements), and we will suggest some changes that we think would make aging more successful for more people.

Third, we will look at older Americans from the viewpoint of those who would be of service to them and suggest an approach to helping that is based on our understanding of what one can do to promote successful aging when working with older people and their families.

Who Are the Aged?

Although it may sound flip, the fact is that we are all "the aging." Aging is a process that begins at birth. In some fields of human life, one gets old quickly. World class gymnasts are usually "washed up" at twenty. On the other hand, in 1987, Sir George Solti, music director of the Chicago Symphony, celebrated his seventy-fifth year with a rigorous conducting schedule. In fact, Sir George has resumed solo appearances at the piano.

We have all known young people who seemed "old." By this, we generally mean that despite their physical youth, they are fixed in their ways and not open to new possibilities and experiences. Conversely, we have also known people who had accumulated a lot of years, but who were still obviously growing and developing. These people are often described as "young for their years." Behind this hopelessly trite phrase lies an important truth—one that we will repeat at every opportunity. Aging is not automatically a wasting away of personal worth. In our society, the tendency among the insensitive is to equate the number of years one has lived with decline. This, we think, is why some consider it remarkable when a young person has an extremely hidebound outlook toward life and an old one seems to be so aware of and charmed by everything that goes on around him or her.

The point that we are aiming at is simply that it is difficult to define just when one becomes old. The answer depends on the frame of reference (for example, gymnastics or music) and the individual.

Our society has handled age rather arbitrarily. Many *rites de passage* are based on age. In most states, one has to be sixteen to get a driver's license. All states have a minimum age at which one can marry with or without parental consent. One must be eighteen to vote, twenty-five to be a member of the House of Representatives, thirty-two to be a member of the Senate, and thirty-five to be president.

With respect to aging, American society regards sixty-five as a significant benchmark. For example, one can retire at sixty-five and receive full Social Security benefits. Until recently, sixty-five was used as a mandatory retirement age in many businesses and governmental positions. As in the case of the other age-based barriers, there is no magic about this one either.

While we must register a protest to the use of any specific year as a line of demarcation between the aging and the "nonaging" (remember that no one is nonaging!), we concede that for our purposes in this chapter, we are stuck with sixty-five because of the way the data are collected.

Size and Distribution of the Aging Population

In this sort of book, it is impossible to provide current figures. First, there is a two-year lag (at least) between the time the figures are collected and when they are reported. Second, figures go out of date between the time a book is written and the time it is actually in use.

We cannot compensate for this problem entirely. Our solution is to try to stick with general trends that are clearly observable over time. Unless noted otherwise, all figures that we use are from the Bureau of the Census' *Statistical Abstract of the United States: 1987* or *Aging America: Trends and Projections*, a publication of the U.S. Senate Special Committee on Aging. Where exact citations are used, we will refer to these sources as the *Statistical Abstract 1987* and *Aging America.*

In 1985, a point halfway between the census years of 1980 and 1990, the U.S. population was approximately 240 million, of whom 28.5 million, or roughly 12%, were sixty-five or older. Just twenty-five years before, in 1960, the percentage of persons sixty-five and over was just over 9%. The Census Bureau estimates that the number of people sixty-five and over will grow to approximately 13% of the population by the year 2000. Clearly, the older population is both growing in numbers and in the percent of the population that those numbers represent.

Further, there has been a remarkable increase in the number of Americans who are seventy-five and older. In 1960, about 5.5 million were seventy-five and over. Twenty-five years later, that number had more than doubled to around 11.5 million.

Of the persons sixty-five and older as of 1985, approximately 60% were female and 40% male. In ethnic terms, approximately 8.2% of Americans sixty-five and over are black, while 2.8% are of Spanish origin (as the Census Bureau puts it). By the year 2000, the Census Bureau predicts that about 8.5% of those sixty-five and over will be black and just under 5% will be of Spanish origin.

Marital Status and Living Arrangements

In 1985, of the 7,259,000 men between sixty-five and seventy-four years of age, approximately 5.2% were single, 81.3% were married, 9.3% were widowed, and 4.2% were divorced. Of the men seventy-five and over, 5.3% were single, 69.3% were married, 22.7% were widowed, and 2.7% were divorced (*Statistical Abstract 1987*, p. 39).

For women between sixty-five and seventy-four years of age, 4.4% were single, 51.1% were married, 38.9% were widowed, and 5.6% were divorced. Women seventy-five and over included 6.2% single, 23.8% married, 67.7% widowed, and 2.4% divorced (*Statistical Abstract 1987*, p. 39).

It is important to note that older women are much more likely to be widows than older men are to be widowers. When one adds up the figures, nearly 50% of the women aged sixty-five to seventy-four are unmarried while only about 19% of the men in that age bracket are not married. For women seventy-five and over, more than three-quarters are unmarried, while only about 31% of men seventy-five and over are unmarried.

The importance of this lies in the increased likelihood of older women to have financial difficulties. Because men have traditionally held higher paying jobs, older women who are alone, whether single, divorced, or widowed, are more likely to have lower incomes. Of course, those women who are widows of men who have left them comfortably fixed may have few money troubles. Some divorcées are well off, and there are women who have never married who have done well. Unfortunately, not all widows have money, many divorcées have financial problems, and many single older women did not have the opportunity to earn large salaries or to save great sums of money. While the poor are a minority among the aged, women are over-represented, particularly those who live alone.

Persons who work with older Americans need to be aware of the greater potential for economic vulnerability among women. At the same time, people whose work brings them into contact with older women are often struck by the recognition of how strong most older women are, both physically and emotionally.

Another way of looking at the circumstances of older people is to examine the data on living arrangements. In 1985, approximately 27 million of the U.S. population who were sixty-five or older lived in households. (*Note:* Earlier we said that the population sixty-five and older was 28.5 million. The discrepancy is simply because about 1.5 million live in institutions, are homeless, or are not accounted for because of sampling errors.) Approximately 30% lived alone, 53% lived with a spouse, 14% lived with other relatives, and 3% lived with nonrelatives.

When blacks and whites are considered separately, some interesting differences are noted. Among whites, 30% lived alone, 55% lived with a spouse, 13% lived with other relatives, and 2% lived with nonrelatives. For blacks, 30% lived alone, only 38% lived with a spouse, 26% lived with other relatives, and 6% lived with nonrelatives. While the percentage of both races who lived alone is virtually identical, fewer blacks sixty-five and over were living with a spouse, twice as many blacks were living with relatives, and three times as many blacks were living with unrelated persons.

The differences are more apparent when both gender and race are taken into consideration. In table 1.1, we have shown these percentages.

Inspection of the table shows that white males are least likely to live alone after age sixty-five, while white females are most likely. It is also important to note that both male and female blacks are more likely to live with relatives than are their white counterparts. Whether this reflects greater importance placed on family support among blacks or simply their relatively disadvantaged economic position is not made clear by these figures.

Table 1.1   Living Arrangements of Persons Sixty-Five Years and Over by Gender and Race.

		Percent Living:		
	Alone	With Spouse	With Relatives	With Nonrelatives
All males	14.7	75.0	7.5	2.9
Whites	14.2	76.8	6.6	2.4
Blacks	29.8	38.3	26.1	5.8
All females	41.1	38.3	18.4	2.1
Whites	41.8	39.5	16.7	2.0
Blacks	36.2	26.4	33.2	4.2

Source: *Statistical Abstract, 1987*, p. 46.

Where Do the Aged Live?

The Census Bureau divides the country into four broad regions. The Northeast includes all of New England, New York, Pennsylvania, and New Jersey. The South includes Maryland, Delaware, West Virginia, Kentucky, Arkansas, Oklahoma, Texas, Louisiana, Mississippi, Alabama, Tennessee, Georgia, Florida, North and South Carolina, and Virginia. The Midwest includes Ohio, Michigan, Indiana, Wisconsin, Illinois, Minnesota, Iowa, Missouri, North and South Dakota, Nebraska, and Kansas. The rest of the country is considered the West.

Of the approximately 28.5 million persons sixty-five and over in 1985, 23% live in the Northeast, 26% live in the Midwest, 34% live in the South, and 17% live in the West. Of course, the validity of this distribution of older Americans is dependent upon acceptance of the regional boundaries used by the Census Bureau. If one looks only at the numbers, the five states with the most persons sixty-five and over are: California, Florida, New York, Pennsylvania, and Texas. It may be more helpful to list the states with the highest proportions of older people: Florida (17.6%), Rhode Island (14.4%), Arkansas (14.3%), Iowa (14.3%), Pennsylvania (14.3%), Missouri (13.7%), South Dakota (13.7%), Nebraska (13.5%), Massachusetts (13.4%), Kansas (13.3%), and West Virginia (13.3%). The states with the lowest proportion of the state's population of persons sixty-five and over include: Alaska (3.2%), Nevada (7.9%), Wyoming (8.3%), Colorado (8.8%), Texas (9.4%), Hawaii (9.4%), New Mexico (9.6%), Louisiana (9.8%), Nevada (9.9%), and Georgia (9.9%) (*Statistical Abstract 1987*, p. 23).

Income

In order to provide a frame of reference in which to discuss the income of older people, it will help to discuss the income of citizens of the United States in general. However, we must warn you that the figures must be interpreted with caution. The income figures in general use are collected by the Census Bureau as part of regular surveys called the Current Population Surveys (CPS). In a book that is concerned with the economics of aging, Schulz (1985, p. 19) notes:

> Income information from surveys like the CPS are [sic] subject to substantial reporting errors by those interviewed. Respondents do not know, remember incorrectly, refuse to answer, or give false information out of anger for fear of government retribution.

In 1985, the personal income of all citizens totaled $3,314,500,000 before taxes. In current 1985 dollars, this comes to an average pretax income of $13,876 for each man, woman, and child in the United States, which is up from $4,051 in 1970. There are, of course, regional differences. Using the regional divisions mentioned earlier, the average income in the Northeast was $15,571. In the Midwest it was $13,519, while the South had $12,570 and the West had $14,740.

Here, again, it is instructive to look at household rather than per capita income. The mean income per household was $27,464. When ethnicity is considered, the average white household had $28,597. Black household income averaged $17,966. Since persons of Spanish origin (who, the Census Bureau tells us, may be members of any race) have now become a sizable segment of the U.S. population, they are receiving official notice. The mean household income among persons of Spanish origin was $21,129 in 1985.

Now let us look at the income of households sixty-five and over. For all U.S. households in which at least one person was over sixty-five, the mean income per household was $18,279 in 1985. For white households, it was $18,790, for blacks it was $12,042, and for persons of Spanish origin, it was $14,045. Clearly, older members of ethnic minorities operate at an economic disadvantage. This is a legacy of the historic income gaps between whites and minorities in the United States. These gaps in the population sixty-five and older are not likely to close until income gaps between younger segments of the population are closed.

Parenthetically, we would like to point out that the overall disadvantaged position of blacks and persons of Spanish origin often seems to lead well-intentioned persons to generalize. Put simply, there is still a tendency among some whites to think that all blacks are alike and that all persons of Spanish origin are pretty much the same.

While it is true that blacks and persons of Spanish origin may have had the nearly universal experience of discrimination, this has not robbed either group of the ability to develop rich and diverse cultures. The helping professionals must look beyond stereotypes and generalizations. There are great individual differences among members of minority groups, and the range of values, tastes, and behaviors is as wide as it is among any collectivity. Although members of ethnic groups are considered as a whole for a number of statistical purposes, they cannot be considered identical for service purposes. Needs and wants will differ with personal circumstances.

The official poverty lines in 1985 were $5,156 for one person and $6,503 for two persons. Looking at the averages, it is clear that most older persons are not in absolute poverty, even members of minority groups, although the relative differences remain.

While it is encouraging to note that poverty among older U.S. citizens has declined to a rate lower than that of the general population (12.6% for persons sixty-five and over versus 14% for citizens in general in 1985), it remains true that a fair number of persons sixty-five and over are officially poor. Approximately 3,456,000 citizens sixty-five and over have incomes below the official poverty line. Here, again, we see differences by gender and ethnicity. Of those who are sixty-five and over and white, 11% are poor. Among blacks, 31.5% of those sixty-five and over are poor, while among those of Spanish origin, 23.9% are officially poor. In households of persons over sixty-five that include a male, the poverty rate is 6%, while in households in which the householder is a woman alone, the poverty rate is 12.1%.

It has been pointed out that the official poverty figures may be misleading in that only cash income is counted in arriving at the definition of poverty. Medical payments through either Medicare or Medicaid are not included, nor is the value of food stamps and subsidized housing. Recognizing this, in 1983 the U.S. Bureau of the Census began to calculate poverty rates using several alternative approaches. At this point, these approaches are used for reporting purposes only. The most conservative alternative approach is the "market value" approach. The market value represents what it would cost to purchase the amount of food, housing, and medical benefits consumed by older citizens. Using this procedure, only about 3% of persons sixty-five and over would be considered living below the poverty level (*Statistical Abstract 1987*, p. 446). However, even if this extremely conservative estimate is used, around three-quarters of a million citizens sixty-five and over—enough to populate the city of Cleveland—remain very poor.

The other side of the coin is revealed when one looks at the figures on wealth. Persons sixty-five to seventy-four years of age have an average net worth in excess of $125,000 (*Statistical Abstract 1987*, p. 451), largely as a consequence of the higher incomes since World War II and the appreciation in real estate. This wealth is not evenly distributed among the aged, of course, but it is instructive to compare persons sixty-five and over with persons aged forty-five to fifty-four—those considered as in the most affluent decade of life (*Statistical Abstract 1987*, p. 451). Fifty-three percent of those sixty-five and over have a savings account, as do 65% of those forty-five to fifty-four. Eighteen percent of those sixty-five and over have a money market account, compared to 12% of those forty-five to fifty-four. Thirty-seven percent of those sixty-five and over have certificates of deposit, compared to 18% of those forty-five to fifty-four. Only 8% of persons sixty-five and over have an Individual Retirement Account (IRA) or Keogh Plan account compared to 25% of persons forty-five to fifty-four. This may merely reflect the relative novelty of the IRA and Keogh Plans, which have only been available in the past few years. Fourteen percent of persons sixty-five and over hold U.S. Savings Bonds, compared to 23% of persons forty-five to fifty-four.

Twenty-one percent of persons sixty-five and over own common stocks, compared with 22% of those forty-five to fifty-four. Only 4% of persons sixty-five and over own corporate and other bonds, but only 3% of persons forty-five to fifty-four own these items. Twenty percent of persons sixty-five and over own real property (in addition to a home), as do 22% of persons forty-five to fifty-four. Seven percent of persons sixty-five and over own a business, compared to 11% of persons forty-five to fifty-four.

These figures do not show how much cash, how many stocks and bonds, or the extent of the property older persons hold in comparison with persons forty-five to fifty-four. They do suggest, however, that there is a certain level of affluence among a fairly sizable number of older people, and that the percentages of older persons with assets is not radically different from that of middle-aged persons. As the "baby boomers" enter the ranks of those sixty-five and over (around the year 2010), many will find themselves very well fixed, both from their own earnings and from inheritances from their relatively more affluent parents.

Education

The older American is better educated than was true just a few years ago. At least, he or she has more formal schooling (this is not the place to engage in an extended discussion of the quality of that education). In 1970, for example, slightly over 50% of Americans in general had four years of high school or more. By 1985, this percentage had grown to just under 74%. As one would expect, the amount of formal education is higher for whites than for either blacks or persons of Spanish origin, but the percentages of persons completing four years of high school or more have increased faster for these ethnic minorities than for whites in recent years.

Among older persons, by 1985, nearly 50% of all Americans age sixty-five or older had had four years of high school or more. One projection suggests that by 1990, the gap between the educational attainment of older Americans and younger Americans will continue to close (*Aging America*, p. 113). This same publication suggests that there are two reasons for this phenomenon. One is the increased educational opportunities that became available after World War II, and the other relates to the lower proportion of immigrants, who have traditionally possessed little formal education, among today's aging population.

The major implication is, we think, that increasingly the older person in this country will be a more discerning consumer of services. We have seen how older people have become much more politically visible in recent years. This is bound to affect both the nature and quality of programs for the aging.

Housing

There are approximately 18 million households of persons sixty-five and over. About 75% live in houses that they own. Almost 80% of these homes are paid for (*Aging America*, p. 116). As a general rule, older people tend to live in the house that they lived in when they were younger. If they remain in good health and their incomes are high enough, this usually is not a problem. Besides, if they need to move, or simply prefer to move, the house can be sold for a significant amount of money, which can be invested in ways that will provide additional income. Therefore, for most older people, housing is not a major problem.

However, there are Americans for whom home ownership is not an advantage. First, for those without sufficient income to maintain the house, there is a good chance that the home will deteriorate and become unsafe. It will also lose value. Second, some older people live in homes that are located in unsafe neighborhoods. As a consequence, their personal mobility is limited by their fears.

About 25% of older Americans who are the primary occupants of households live in rental property. Here again, if one has enough money to rent a decent place, it is no problem. However, for the older individual with a limited amount of disposable income, finding a good house or apartment will be difficult.

There is limited public housing available. Currently, approximately 373,000 units are available for rental by persons sixty-two and over who meet an income criterion. This is a resource that, like public housing in general, is not expanding appreciably. While public housing has generally come into disfavor, it has worked well for older tenants. As this is being written, however, national policy appears to favor a voucher system for rentals to low-income people, rather than the building of additional public housing units. Even if there were a complete reversal in national policy, it would take years for additional units to get into the "pipeline," so the outlook for public housing for older people is very limited over the short term. Whether this is good or bad, of course, depends on one's ideological point of view.

Employment

About three million Americans sixty-five and over are employed. These people represent a little less than 3% of the labor force. Traditionally, retirement at age sixty-five was mandatory, but for governmental jobs and private jobs in which governmental contracts are involved, the mandatory retirement age is now seventy.

We will say more about retirement in later chapters. All we want to say here is that many older Americans continue to work beyond age sixty-five. While it is too soon to consider it a trend, there is an effort on the part of some employers to hire older people as part-time workers. McDonald's, for example, has a program to hire older workers since they are unable to hire enough young people to staff their fast-food outlets.

On the other hand, many older citizens prefer to retire earlier than is necessary. Currently, about 40% of American workers choose to take early retirement. As we shall explain in more detail later, one receives a reduced Social Security benefit at age sixty-two. However, many persons, because they have savings and good pension benefits, elect to retire early.

Health

Persons sixty-five and over spend about twice as much on medical care than the general population does, and they spend about three times as many days in the hospital. They have over three times the cardiovascular problems of younger people. And older persons have proportionately more physical limitations than younger persons do.

On the other hand, most Americans sixty-five and over consider their health to be good. While it is generally true that the older one gets, the less healthy one is, the point at which one's physical condition becomes severely limiting is much later now than it used to be. We now see many people who are vigorous up into their eighties—something that was comparatively rare sixty years ago.

In terms of mental health, older people do not have as many problems as younger people do. However, the problems that older persons have are apt to be severe, particularly those problems that affect cognitive functioning.

Demographic Characteristics ───────────

Americans are living longer. Most of them have more money than their parents, believe their health to be good, have higher education, own their own homes and choose to retire early. While the picture of most older Americans is positive, there are disturbing aspects. There are still poor older Americans, and there remain status differentials due to race, ethnicity, and gender.

Additional Subpopulations ─────────────

There are a number of other subpopulations that we want to call to your attention. We think that it is important to be sensitive to the special needs that they may have.

Asian-Americans

Great cultural diversity exists among those persons classified as Asian-Americans. Asian culture is extremely complex, and there are great differences among Chinese-Americans, Japanese-Americans, Korean-Americans, and others. Some Asian-Americans have been in the United States for many years and are quite thoroughly acculturated. Others, those from Vietnam, for example, may be relatively new and will have radically different circumstances from those with a longer history in this country.

As of the 1980 census there were about a quarter million persons age sixty-five and older of Asian or Pacific island descent living in the United States (AARP, no date; this document is the source for all the data on Asian-Americans). Most are concentrated in California, Hawaii, and Washington, but many others live in the New York and Chicago areas or in Texas.

There are, unlike other ethnic groups, more men than women among the aged. Most men sixty-five and over are married, while most women are widowed. Only 19% of the Asian-American aged live alone. However, it will probably be difficult for the Asian-American woman who lives alone. Asian women traditionally did not work outside the home. Consequently, these women are more likely to have language problems and be isolated from others in the community.

Although many older Asian-Americans are well educated, the newer arrivals tend to be below the average in formal education. More continue to work after age sixty-five than is true for whites, probably due to their need for income rather than anything else, since the median income for Asian-Americans is significantly lower than for whites. Despite the income differences, the percentage of Asian-Americans who were officially poor in 1980 was about the same as it was for whites.

There are few data on the health status of Asian-Americans, but the AARP reports that there is a tendency among some to rely on folk medicines and to distrust Western medicine.

Native Americans

Stuart and Rathbone-McCuan (1988) have studied the position of the American Indian elderly in the United States. The material in this section is abstracted from their work. They note that although the number of elderly Indian Americans increased from around 16,000 to 75,000 between 1930 and 1980, their proportion among the American Indian population has remained at about 5%. Stuart and Rathbone-McCuan observe that these people have the shorter life expectancy associated with the relative poverty that is characteristic of minority groups in the United States.

A little over one-third of American Indians live on reservations or on traditional tribal lands. Because of the dispersion of Indians from traditional areas and because there are difficulties in deciding who is an Indian, hard statistics are difficult to obtain. However, the National Indian Council on Aging estimated (in 1981) that approximately 61% of the Indian elderly lived in poverty and had severe health problems. These problems were especially severe for older Indians who lived on reservations. Reservation Indians aged fifty-five and above, for example, had levels of health impairment not usually seen in the general population until ten years later.

Since American Indians aged sixty-five and over constitute less than 1% of the older population in the United States, most service professionals will see few of them, unless they work in states with large Indian populations. We have included the American Indians in this discussion primarily to call attention to what must be the worst examples of both policy failure and faulty service delivery in the entire Western world. Stuart and Rathbone-McCuan detail the history of inconsistent federal policy, the reluctance of states to provide legitimate benefits to Indian citizens, and a national lack of concern for them in general and the elderly in particular. There is little coordination of services and, apparently, a good deal of bureaucratic infighting about who should do what for whom. There is an implicit lesson here that services for older people must be planned with some kind of a sense of what the consumer wants and can use, and must take into account the varied characteristics of the clientele.

The Very Old

We mentioned earlier that the population aged seventy-five and over is increasing. We want to extend that discussion as a separate issue in order to highlight the population that is eighty-five and over. In the United States, the population eighty-five and over has grown faster than any other age segment. It will continue to do so in the next century. "Between 1984 and 2050, the population aged eighty-five and over is expected to jump from about 1 percent to over 5 percent of the total population and from 9 percent to 24 percent of the sixty-five-plus population" (*Aging America* 1985, p. 15). These older people will probably be mostly women. Since this age group is more likely to have health problems—and may have outlived their savings and pensions—they constitute a policy challenge for the future.

Gays and Lesbians

Berger (1984) has provided the most useful information about the status of older gays and lesbians. Service providers, Berger argues, need to be better informed and less inclined to stereotype the homosexual. The primary thing that service providers need to understand, according to Berger, is that self-acceptance as a homosexual often is not "integrated" until later life, and this adjustment may be difficult and may complicate other aspects of the homosexual's life. Otherwise, it was his conclusion that "older homosexuals have much in common with older heterosexuals" (p. 61), and that while the recluse does exist, most do not end up "isolated and depressed," but function "in networks of friends, lovers, family, and community institutions." The major problems, he found, were discrimination in housing and employment.

Berger believes that older gays and lesbians generally need "the same services as all older adults: health care, income maintenance, transportation, social and recreational outlets and emotional support" (p. 61). He recognizes that, because mainstream social agencies have not been able or willing to offer specialized services to the aging homosexual, most services will be offered by homosexual groups in the foreseeable future.

Components of Successful Aging

This is not a text in gerontology—the study of aging. Rather, it is intended to aid helping professionals in their work with older people—to promote successful aging. Even so, we recognize the necessity of having a theoretical orientation about what aging is. We could not conceive of successful aging without some notion of what it is that one is to be successful at!

A fundamental theoretical problem was originally posed by Bernice Neugarten (1981) and is still unsolved: from a developmental point of view, it is not possible to separate the characteristics of aging as a process from the social and cultural conditions in which aging takes place. At the other end of life, the characteristics of the developing child are relatively easy to see. He or she has growth characteristics, physical, mental, and social, that are clearly developmental. Although child development is influenced by culture, developmental processes are relatively easy to look at, independent of culture. Clearly, the goal of child development is an adult organism. To what developmental end does the aging process (whatever it is) point? How should aging persons look when they are successfully getting on with the business of aging? Or, is it even legitimate to think of aging persons in terms of development at all? To some, aging represents not development, but decline, as is the case with fruit or vegetables. After a certain prime period, the apple begins to wrinkle and lose flavor, the potato to rot. Is this analogous to the human condition, in that the only possible "development" is decline?

Part of the problem is that there has been a great deal more research in the development of the young. We are still trying to ask the right questions about adult development and have not yet accumulated enough data to provide an adequate developmental theory. This is not to say that there are no theories about aging, because there are. However, the most prominent are not developmental theories. They are largely sociocultural theories that deal primarily with the meaning of aging in a cultural contest; they do not integrate the biological and physiological realms very well. We will summarize them briefly here and then we will outline the premises on which this book is written.

Activity Theory

Activity theory is Neugarten's name for the notion that "except for changes in biology and health, older people are the same as middle-aged people, with essentially the same psychological and social needs"

(Neugarten, 1981, p. 225). The idea here is that aging is an extension of one's previous life and differs only in that one is physically showing signs of wear that limit one's activities. In response, society tends to withdraw from the aging person, even though the aging person wants to continue to participate. Successful aging, in this context, consists of staying active and continuing to live as a middle-aged person as long as possible.

Disengagement Theory

Largely the creation of Elaine Cumming and her colleagues, disengagement theory embodies the notion that as people age, both they and the society mutually disengage from each other. Gradually, as people age, suggests the theory, they participate less actively in the society as a whole. They retire from work and curtail their other activities. From the point of view of society, this is functional, since the disengagement of older persons provides room for younger persons. Thus, disengagement is considered advantageous for both the individual and society. The person who has aged successfully disengages with a sense of accomplishment and satisfaction. The person who has not developed a sense of accomplishment has trouble disengaging and may try to hang on, like an athlete past his or her prime. This seems analogous to Erikson's notion that the person who has satisfactorily resolved the last life crisis of integrity versus despair is the person who has successfully aged.

The Aging as a Subculture

Arnold Rose (1965) defined a subculture as something that begins to develop when a set of people associate with each other more than they associate with others. A fully developed subculture, he said, comes about when the persons have a mutual relationship in which all have an important stake and when other people exclude them from significant interaction. Rose found evidence for the development of an aging subculture in several trends that included the growing number of older people, the tendency for them to segregate themselves in "retirement communities," the increase in retirement and the resultant disengagement from work and work-related activities and relationships, and the tendency for the older and younger generations to live separately.

Rose acknowledged that participation in the aging subculture varies from person to person, and that many older people continue to participate in the larger culture in varying degrees. However, Rose believed that over time older people begin to think of themselves differently and to develop a group identification. Rose postulated the subcultural theory primarily as a framework for research and not as a concept having any normative implications. However, insofar as the theory describes reality, it captures the real position of some older persons in American society. It can be inferred that successful aging, if the aged in fact constitute a subculture, would involve full identification with one's fellow aged and the acceptance of subcultural norms.

Aging as a Social Definition

Levin and Levin (1980) took the radical position that the aging can best be understood as a powerless minority group and that all theories of aging follow Ryan's notion of "blaming the victim" for his or her problems. To Levin and Levin, what gerontologists do is to study older people and identify their characteristics. They then show how those characteristics result in problems, thus blaming the victim for the problem in the first place.

It is the Levins' position that the difficulties of growing old are "as much the result of social as of biological forces." They believe that the problem is misnamed and that the real problem is with the young and their attitudes. The remedy, of course, is to focus on the characteristics of society that discriminate against the aged. Levin and Levin quote Rosow, who believes that what is needed is "a basic re-ordering of our national aspirations and values" because anything less would only be treatment of symptoms.

Clearly, Levin and Levin write out of the radical tradition. Their real target appears to be the capitalist economic system. Consequently, they have no explanation for aging other than an ideological one that traces all personal and social difficulties to the existing social order. Their alternative to "victim blaming" is "system blaming."

We cite their argument not because we find it generally helpful, but because there is some truth in recognizing that when there are things perceived as problematic in any society, part of the cause usually lies in the way the social order works. Therefore, part of the solution involves changes in the way that things work. This does not require a wholesale change in the social system, however.

The variety of approaches to the meaning of aging reminds us of John Godfrey Saxe's poem about the six blind men who went to see an elephant. Each touched a different part of the elephant and believed that his experience was the definitive one. We do not intend to trivialize the theories that have been advanced by making this comparison. Just as there was some truth in the experience of each blind man, there is some truth in each theory. But none can be adopted to the exclusion of the others.

Our Position

Some older persons seem to be understood best in terms of activity theory. That is, for them, their old age is an extension of middle age, and they are able to carry on very much as they had earlier. Service to and on behalf of these people will be aimed at providing them with those resources that enable them to live as they have chosen for as long as they can.

Others can be understood as involved in the process of disengagement from their level of social interaction. For example, as mentioned earlier, many people choose early retirement when they don't have to because they want to do other things that are of personal importance to them. Service to these people will focus on assisting them to disengage smoothly and to find the resources to carry on as they wish, as far as this is possible.

Some aspects of the lives of older people can best be understood in the subcultural frame of reference, that is, in terms of generational identification and mutuality of interest. There is nothing inherently wrong in the notion that older people may identify themselves as a group and develop subcultural norms. In working with older persons, helping professionals need to recognize the subcultural aspects of the life of the aging.

Finally, while we tend to think that Levin and Levin have overstated their case and that the aged cannot fairly be understood primarily as objects of discrimination, these researchers do have a point. There are issues and instances when it is clear that some of the old in some places and at some times are victims of discrimination and insensitivity. Successful aging, in these situations, requires that helping professionals assist older persons and groups of older persons who are challenging those unenlightened aspects of the social order that are detrimental to legitimate human aspirations.

We think that there is much good sense in Neugarten's position. After reviewing the research on personality change in old age, she concluded that "given a relatively supportive social environment, older persons, like younger ones, will choose the combinations of activities that offer them the most ego-involvement and that are most consonant with their long-established value patterns and self-concepts" (Neugarten, 1981, p. 226).

We think that successful aging involves two basic things: (1) the freedom to choose among alternatives; and (2) a supportive social environment in which alternatives exist. This is an idealistic moral position, and we do not apologize for it. One must have a vision to guide his or her activity. These two things can be broken into five components. First, the successful older person must have enough money to enjoy a decent level of existence. While it is not necessary that everyone be wealthy, we believe that older people should not have to be desperately poor, but should have enough to permit a level of living that allows a healthy and varied diet, a clean, safe place to live, comfortable and decent clothing, good quality health care, and the desired kind and amount of recreational activity.

Second, successful aging depends upon one's health. While service providers and public policy makers obviously cannot wave a wand and create good health for older persons, they can provide a level of care that offers health services consistent with prevailing medical standards.

Third, successful aging involves a positive state of mental health. This, too, cannot be mandated by any social institution, but we believe that this country has the resources to provide a decent level of preventive and therapeutic services consistent with good practice. Efforts also need to be made to educate the general public to recognize that mental symptoms are not the inevitable result of old age, but signs that one is ill and needs treatment. When treatment is needed, it should be provided in clinics and hospitals that meet licensing standards and by professionals who take a positive view of aging.

Fourth, the person who ages successfully needs a safe environment in which to live and one that provides a decent level of services that the older person may use as he or she chooses.

Finally, successful aging includes the opportunity for satisfying relationships with one's family and friends. The older person should be protected from abuse by other family members. Further, older persons ought to be able to maintain meaningful friendships; they should not be forced into lives of isolation.

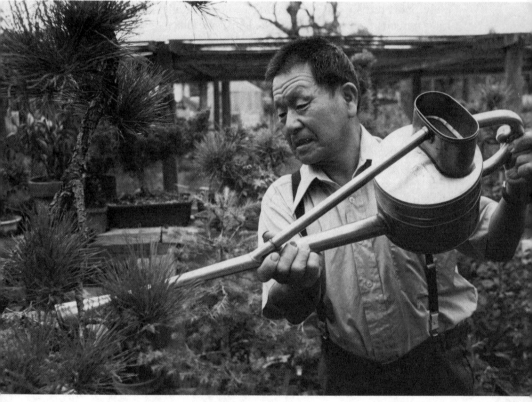

© Marianne Gontarz

2

Perspectives on Older Persons

Our ability to work successfully with older persons to improve the quality of their lives is heavily influenced by the way we view old age and older persons. If, for example, we see old age as a time of inevitable isolation, decline, and decay, it will be difficult for us to be motivated to help a widow to find new friends and interests and to improve her health status. If, on the other hand, we believe that growth and change are possible regardless of age, we will be motivated to help even very old persons articulate what they want and develop plans to get it. It is important for people considering a career in aging to examine carefully what they believe old age can and should be. Such an examination should help ensure that their own beliefs, attitudes, and values are consistent with helping older persons achieve the most satisfying lives possible. In this chapter we discuss some perspectives on old age and the elderly that we believe have a strong positive influence on the kinds of helping relationships we can develop with older persons.

Older Persons Are Unique Individuals

It is hard to spend much time with older people without being struck by how different they are from one another. While it is important for anyone working with the elderly to have summary information about the characteristics of older people as a whole, it is equally important to be aware of the diversity that exists among them. A good argument can be made for the statement that the elderly population is more heterogeneous than any other population.

Differences arise from a number of sources, including the characteristics with which people are born. Men and women are different, and historically they have been treated differently. These differences influence how men and women experience both physiological and social aging. They also result in the different meanings that men and women attribute to the circumstances of late life.

Women, for example, are viewed as "old" and unattractive at an earlier chronological age than men. This "double aging standard" which Sontag (1972) described, may lead women to attempt to disguise their ages to a far greater degree than men. It may also lead men to believe older women are less desirable as companions than younger women. Married women are far more likely to lose a spouse through death than are men. There is some reason to believe that because women are aware of this likelihood and anticipate widowhood in old age, the transition to widowhood is easier for them than it is for men. Although not much is known about sex differences in adjustment to retirement, there is reason to expect that retirement may have different consequences and meanings for men than for women.

Another source of difference is racial or ethnic background. Those who work with the elderly must be aware, for example, that people who are white generally had more favorable circumstances throughout their lifetimes than did blacks. A lifetime of low earnings based on racial or ethnic discrimination in employment can result in lower life expectancy and poverty in old age. In addition to the effects of discrimination, diversity by racial or ethnic group may be reflected in different preferences for family involvement in old age, different attachment to cultural symbols, and different orientations to death. It is important for those who anticipate working with elderly populations different from their own to become as familiar as possible with these populations' distinctive traditions and expectations. To avoid doing so is to risk poor communication, considerable misunderstanding, and social injustice. In addition to the differences that have their roots in birth characteristics, it is important to recognize that each older individual, regardless of gender or race, has experienced a special series of events (or life course) that contributes to his or her uniqueness in old age.

Imagine all the babies born in your hometown in 1920. As babies, they probably all tended to be pretty similar. They ate, slept, and cried. They liked to have clean diapers and to be cuddled. As these babies grew and experienced more of the world, however, they began to have different experiences. They may have gone to different schools and churches and all were influenced by different family situations. They were affected differently by the physical environment, including weather, pollution, and geographic features. As they grew to adulthood, some married and some did not. Some experienced great success in their careers; others had trouble scraping by. Each individual developed his or her own way of dealing with the challenges and opportunities that life presented. If the survivors of this group should meet today, they would certainly be far different from one another than they were as infants in 1920. It is thus foolhardy to approach older persons with the notion that "all older people are pretty much alike," if for no other reason than the length of time available to promote diversity.

Yet another source of diversity in old age is age itself. If we define the aged as "everyone sixty years old or older," we mask the fact that we have identified at least two (and possibly three) generations of people. This has recently been highlighted by a distinction made between the young-old (relatively healthy, active, well-off individuals who are the youngest elderly chronologically) and the old-old (persons in frail health with fewer economic resources who are older chronologically than the young-old). It is not uncommon to encounter families in which young-old members have responsibility for providing care and assistance to old-old members. Differences might be expected between the "younger" and "older" elderly not only on the basis of health status, functional abilities, and economic status, but also on outlook toward life.

The reason for these differences is that events in the outside world influence the courses that lives take. Further, these events are likely to have affected people differently, depending on how old the person was when the event occurred. For example, it is generally acknowledged that the worst year of the Great Depression was 1933. Millions of Americans were unemployed, and many families could not afford decent shelter. People who achieved age sixty in 1988 were five years old in 1933; people who achieved age eighty in 1988 were twenty in 1933. A man who was twenty in 1933 is unlikely to have gone to college unless his parents were very well-to-do. He is likely to have delayed marriage and had fewer children. He may also have developed a distinctive set of attitudes and political orientations arising from the economic hardship that he experienced as a young man about to start out in the world. These experiences from his youth can well be expected to have long-term consequences that manifest themselves in old age. One consequence of having fewer children than people who turned twenty earlier and later than he did is that he has fewer children to whom he might turn for support in old age. A consequence of his inability to continue his education is that his lifetime earnings were lower than they might have been otherwise, affecting both his ability to save for his old age and the amount of his eventual retirement pension. By contrast, the man who was age five at the worst of the Depression may have only faint recollections of the economic hardships that his family experienced. By the time he turned twenty, it was 1948, a period of economic prosperity. He is considerably more likely to have gone to college and to have found a good job at the outset of his career. Moreover, he entered the childbearing years at a time when big families were encouraged. As a result of these differences in the experience of historical events, it is likely that both his objective circumstances in old age and his attitudes and values will be different than those of the elderly person twenty years his senior.

A further point to note in discussing the individuality of the older person is that people's wants and needs do not necessarily change because they have grown old. As we noted earlier, the growing number of older persons in our midst has generated considerable attention. Numerous articles and books have been written about the "older population," discussing everything from older persons' religious preferences to their use of leisure time. These are then often compared with general characteristics of younger age groups and differences are found, leaving the impression that older persons are a category somehow different in important respects from the rest of us. One might even be led to the belief that becoming old results in significant changes in what individuals want and what interests them.

In fact, radical changes in interests or wants rarely occur with advanced age. While we may take on new activities and interests at an advanced age, most of us pursue into later life the interests and abilities that are consistent with those we developed in our younger years. Older persons' current interests and abilities have been shaped by their own unique life histories and their values about what they regard as important ways to spend their time. As is the case with younger people, the old take pride in their accomplishments; when they invest time in a project, they want it to be something of meaning. For this reason, we are skeptical of activity programs at nursing homes or other places when the primary purpose is to keep people busy. Workers who encourage people to pursue meaningful long-standing interests (crocheting an afghan for an expected grandchild, raising vegetables to be canned or shared with others, volunteering time to help an illiterate adult learn to read) and offer opportunities for older people to pursue their own choices in new activities take a far more sensible and respectful approach than do those who act on their own assumptions about what older people ought to be doing with their time.

The central point of this discussion is that it is important to approach the aged person as an individual, shaped by circumstances of birth, the historical period at which he or she experienced different life events, and the individual choices made during the course of that life. While information about the "average" older person can be helpful, it is important to remember in dealing with individual older persons that their current situations and total life experiences may be very different from the statistical norm. Each person should be approached and evaluated on his or her own terms with the understanding that an aged person's unique life history has contributed substantially to who he or she is today.

Older Persons Are Survivors

A central premise in the helping professions is to build on the client's strengths. This means that when a person is having trouble, it is usually helpful to emphasize the successes the person has had and the skills and resources the person has used in the past to resolve problems. An important thing to remember in building on strengths is that aged people are survivors. To be blunt, they would not have lived to old age unless they were able to muster some skills and resources that helped them stay alive. While it may be helpful for an older person to refocus energies and apply skills in different ways to resolve current problems, most older persons have survived through a number of trying life experiences and have a deep reservoir of past successes in problem resolution to draw upon.

This perspective is important for the professional for at least two reasons. First, it draws attention to the positive aspects of the older person's life history. It is helpful for professionals who tend to view the people with whom they work as dependent and "in need" to see the other, resourceful side of the person who is now requesting their assistance. The emphasis on survivorship and strengths can be instructive to the young person who is apprehensive about his or her own personal aging. It is not uncommon for young professionals to be amazed at the stories they hear when attempting to identify problem-solving skills used by older persons in the past. Often they gain renewed respect for aged persons from whom they previously thought they had nothing to learn.

A second reason why the survivor perspective may be helpful for the young professional is that it suggests that the older person is likely to survive unintended mistakes that the professional may make in the helping process. Some beginning professionals are afraid that their attempts at intervention will not meet with all the success they hope for and will have disastrous consequences for the persons they are trying to serve. Most of the time this is not the case. Of course, this discussion is not meant to suggest that it is all right to take a sloppy approach to work with older persons. Quite the contrary! It is simply intended to highlight the fact that a person who has survived seventy or eighty years of living is likely to survive an unintended minor mistake made by a service provider. With competent supervision, the worker usually has an opportunity to recognize the mistake and remedy it.

Older Persons Are Responsible, Capable Beings

We take the position that, barring severe mental illness, older persons should be viewed as capable of making responsible choices affecting their own destinies. Just as is the case at earlier points in the life course, late life presents choices both about actions that one may take or fail to take (entering a nursing home, applying for food stamps) and about how one will interpret, or give meaning to, life circumstances. People are constantly in the process of creating their own lives through these choices, and the process does not cease in old age. In fact, it can be argued that the significance of being able to make free choices is even greater in old age than it is in younger years. In contrast to the young, older people are keenly aware of what has been called the "foreshortened life perspective" (Butler and Lewis, 1982). While the young have time to remedy mistakes and a seemingly endless future in which to make new choices to alter their lives, the elderly do not enjoy the luxury of time. Because opportunities for experiences in the future are limited, older persons are often particularly careful about the choices they make and devote their energies only to those things that seem most important.

Making important new choices in late life can be one outcome of the life review process first described by Butler (1963). Butler notes that older persons tend to spend considerable time thinking and (sometimes) talking about the courses their lives have taken in an effort to come to some understanding of the meaning of it all. From this perspective, old age is not necessarily a time of calm, contentment, and relaxation. For many, the life review process entails confronting past disappointment, resentment, and unresolved anger, as well as accomplishments and satisfactions. It thus involves making choices about how one will evaluate the totality of one's life near its end. Usually, the evaluation made during the life review is positive, resulting in a decision that the life lived represents the best one could have done under the circumstances. One outcome, however, can be a choice to right the wrongs of the past in an effort to make peace with self and others before it is too late. In such cases, acting upon late life choices (for example, mending a broken relationship with a sibling) can take on paramount importance.

Not all life reviews have positive outcomes. The professional needs to be particularly careful in working with an older person whose evaluation appears to be resulting in a decision that his or her life has been misspent and is thus not worth living. For these individuals, the "logical" choice often appears to be suicide. Depression and late life suicide are discussed in detail in chapter 5. Counseling with older persons contemplating suicide involves both helping them see the courses their lives have taken from new perspectives and focusing on the future. The intent is that they can come to positive resolutions of their life reviews and reject the option of suicide.

The view of older persons as responsible beings, capable of making their own choices and affecting their own destinies, has other implications. Many adults have a tendency to view older persons as diminished humanity. This is particularly likely if an older person has impaired hearing, cannot drive, needs assistance with dressing, or is in some other way dependent on others' help. Some people begin to look upon such older persons as if they were children. Not only do they provide the assistance needed, but they begin to "teach" dependency by taking over tasks the older person can perform, including decision-making tasks. Well-meaning adult children of the elderly have been known to attempt a kind of role reversal in which they try to "parent" their parents. They go beyond the kind of friendly counsel that adults share with other adults to telling their parents they may no longer drive, that they must apply for services from a social welfare agency, or that they may not marry! Social service workers are not immune from the tendency to treat older persons as if they were children. It is not unusual for professionals to make decisions "in the client's best interest" without consulting the mentally alert but physically impaired older person on whose behalf they are supposedly working. It is our position that it is totally inappropriate for professionals or family members to behave in this manner. Attempts to infantilize are likely to lead to resentment and/or increased dependency on the part of the older person. Neither result contributes to successful aging.

One additional point needs to be raised in a discussion of older persons and the choices they make. Late life can present opportunities for greater freedom of choice than is perceived possible in younger years. This statement may seem paradoxical because we are accustomed to hearing that aging limits, rather than expands, choices. It is true that poor physical health, lack of financial resources, and the patronizing behavior of others often severely limit older persons' freedom. At the same time, freedom from previously held responsibilities can be very liberating.

Older couples whose children have recently left home often express a sense of relief. Not only do they have more money and more time to spend as they please, but they often feel "freer" to be themselves. Because they do not see their children as much as they did, their need to constantly be on their best behavior "to set a good example" is eliminated. Now, what harm is done if the house is not tidied every day or if people want to eat only chocolate cake for dinner?

The same type of freedom is seen after people retire. Fear of social consequences often prevents many people from expressing what they really think on a number of issues. Older people are often better able than younger ones to speak out, because they are less vulnerable to most forms of retaliation. A retired person, for example, cannot be fired if he or she is critical of shoddy merchandise or poor service work. A younger person might be reluctant to be critical, since the business being criticized may be owned by a friend of his or her boss. This may explain why older persons are often the most vocal consumers and citizens: they know that they have less to lose.

Learning, Growth, and Change

One of the most destructive myths about old age is that the elderly are set in their ways and incapable of learning, growth, and change. A large body of experimental research in gerontological psychology suggests that this is simply not the case. When motivated to learn, and when given sufficient time, older persons are just as able to learn new things as are people in any other age group. For many, a life change such as retirement, the emptying of the nest, or even widowhood provides the stimulus for developing new outlooks, lifestyles, and activities, all of which involve learning. While most new learning occurs informally, increasing numbers of older persons are taking advantage of formal educational opportunities. Some seek information and skills pertaining directly to issues concerning old age. They may attend programs offered through senior centers and the American Association of Retired Persons on topics such as defensive driving, financial management, and retirement planning. Others are attracted to Elderhostel and similar programs that bring older adults together to study topics ranging from calligraphy to computers. Still others avoid the age-segregated programs and enroll in adult basic education, college courses, or in continuing education programs offered to the entire community. Our older population is becoming increasingly well educated, and we can expect the demands for learning opportunities in late life to expand accordingly.

Many helping professionals have refused to take on elderly persons as clients under the mistaken belief that substantial change in later life is impossible. After all, if one believes that older persons' personalities and behavior are fixed for life, regardless of their motivation to change or the professional's interventive skills, developing a helping relationship is pointless. This mistaken belief has resulted in many older persons being denied the help they desired and from which they could have benefited.

The helping professional must strenuously avoid the temptation to stereotype the older person as uninterested in learning or incapable of growth and change. When older persons seek help, it is usually because they know they must learn new things in order to improve the quality of their lives. As a result, the helping professional often finds him- or herself in the role of guide or teacher. The "new things to be learned" might include how to identify leisure pursuits that will add meaning to empty hours, how to cope with a spouse suffering from Alzheimer's disease, how to manage on a restricted diet, or how to redevelop a positive self-image following an amputation. Opportunities that the professional can provide include group participation (see chapter 10) or individualized therapy, counseling, or teaching. Regardless of modality, the helping professional who offers hope and conveys a belief that the older person can learn and change in the way desired is more likely to help the older person achieve his or her goals than the one who assumes that the potential for learning and change in old age is limited.

Older Persons Are Members of Families

Virtually all older persons have, at one time or another, lived in a family setting and been heavily influenced by family relationships. Further, the vast majority of older persons are currently in close contact with at least some family members, most often spouse, children, and siblings. As increasing attention has been focused on the problems and concerns of the elderly, however, these facts have often been forgotten. Professionals have been rightly concerned about the isolated elderly who live alone with no visible family ties, and people who come to the attention of health and social service agencies are often viewed as individual "cases" rather than as members of family networks. Since the older person is often "seen" (or treated) as an individual, the tendency can be to minimize the influence family members may have on the situation unless the older person explicitly mentions his or her kin.

Nevertheless, for the vast majority of older persons, relationships with family members are extremely important and must be taken into account in planning and making interventions. Despite prevailing myths, very few older persons are "dumped" into nursing homes or otherwise abandoned by their families. For those who are married (70 to 80 percent of older men and 25 to 50 percent of older women, depending on age), the spouse is the major source of social contact and support. Over 80 percent of older persons who have living children report seeing at least one child once a week or more often. Although both older persons and adult children prefer to maintain separate households if possible, members of both generations expect frequent contact and provide support and assistance to one another when needed. For a number of older persons, a sibling is the closest family member and can be extremely helpful when assistance is needed.

The willingness of family members to help older people who are in need should not be underestimated. Although a variety of programs has emerged in recent years to assist older persons with health and other problems, most of the help given to older persons comes from family members. In fact, family members often work so hard to help older relatives that they put their own mental and physical health at risk. Professionals need to be aware of the complex pressures that caring for dependent elders can create. Considerable strain and negative feelings are reported among family members who give care to infirm elders. Those receiving the care may also feel the quality of their relationships with care-giving kin threatened as they become increasingly dependent. In a small but alarming number of cases, dependency in old age appears to precipitate physical and mental abuse of the elderly by the "care givers." Measures to prevent these negative outcomes (including education of the care givers about dependency in old age and the use of support groups) are discussed in chapter 12. At this point, we want to note that intervention plans for dependent elders who have family should take into account the willingness and capability of those family members to assist.

Of course, the importance of family relationships for older persons goes beyond the family as a source of help in times of need. For most of us, families are the context within which our values and attitudes develop and are maintained. Not surprisingly, it is common for older people to reflect back on their own parents and grandparents for models about how to (or how not to) approach their own aging. In this sense, even family members who died long ago can be an important influence on how people behave in old age. Proceeding in the other direction, older persons often express a desire to leave something of importance to younger generations. They may do considerable planning concerning how their possessions will be distributed after their deaths. They are concerned about their children and grandchildren and whether they were successful in passing along important values to those who will survive them. For many, continuity of self through these new generations can be a source of comfort in the face of death's inevitability.

Many Problems of Older Persons Are Not of Their Making

Throughout this text we emphasize that many of the problems people have in aging "successfully" have their roots in inadequate societal arrangements. Age discrimination in employment frustrates the efforts of an older man who would like to earn extra income after retirement. Reimbursement policies for health care (which tend to pay more for care provided in institutions) make it very difficult for severely disabled older persons to receive the medical care they need while remaining at home. Limitations in eligibility for the Medicaid program can impoverish a well spouse trying to maintain his or her mate in a nursing home. Many communities have been developed with the assumption that every adult can drive an automobile, thereby hampering the mobility of elderly persons who are unable to drive. Despite these and other obvious structural barriers to successful aging, helping professionals are frequently seduced by the tendency to blame the victim. Victim blaming involves the notion that the problem is located in the individual rather than in the society. Somehow the person experiencing difficulties must change; then the problem will be resolved. This is a tempting perspective, because of the belief that it is easier to change a single older person than it is to change social and physical environments that cause problems for that older person.

Professionals should assess each situation carefully. While in some cases it is, indeed, the older person who must change to improve his or her life, in others the problem has its root in societal arrangements. We believe that workers in the field of aging have a twofold task. One part of this task is to acknowledge (both to ourselves and to the people with whom we are working) that barriers like age discrimination and inadequate health care arrangements exist, while at the same time helping older persons live the best lives possible in the current situation. The other part (discussed in chapter 11) involves working to create an environment more conducive to successful aging for today's older people and those of the future. The important point to bear in mind is that not all problems aged persons have can be fully and satisfactorily resolved at the individual level. In some cases, the best we may be able to do is help the older person live within constraints imposed by others and make the best choices possible from the alternatives available.

Older Persons and the Formal Helping System

The needs and problems of older persons have become the focus of considerable attention in recent years. This attention has resulted in the development of a large number of programs and resources aimed at alleviating older persons' problems and providing greater opportunities for them to participate in community life. At the same time, however, it has led to the mistaken impression that all older persons are in need of special programs and services if they are to live their lives satisfactorily. Unfortunately, needs are frequently defined from the perspective of the agency offering the service rather than from that of the older person who is the intended beneficiary of the service.

The authors have known professionals who take the position, for example, that an older person who lives alone "needs" the socialization experiences that participation in senior citizens center activities can provide. Such professionals have strenuously recruited older persons to join senior center activities, only to find that potential recruits were living perfectly happy lives and that the prospect of joining a senior center was not in the least appealing.

In other cases, professionals doing outreach work have found seniors not getting benefits they had requested and to which they were entitled. These seniors had previously applied for services but found, when they became "clients," that their needs, wishes, and dignity were not respected. Or they learned that what they had to go through to receive the service was so complicated or inconvenient that they were better off doing without. They had decided that the costs of receiving the service far outweighed the benefits.

We believe that health and social service agencies should make strong efforts to widely publicize the services they offer. Special efforts may need to be made to ensure that older persons who might want to use the services are aware of their existence. Agency policies and procedures should also be reviewed and revised periodically to ensure that they make it as simple and convenient for older persons to use services as possible. Every effort should be made to see to it that personnel at all levels of the organization respect the comfort, wishes, and dignity of those making use of services. Having made these efforts, however, professionals need to recognize that there are many older persons (including some who may appear to "need" services) who do not want to become clients. Unless there is good reason to doubt the mental competence of the person to whom services are offered, her or his wishes must be respected.

Success May Mean Slowing Deterioration

We have spoken a great deal in this chapter about the ability of older persons to grow and change and to make decisions that can substantially improve the quality of their lives. We believe it is important for professionals to assume this perspective and help older persons live the best lives possible. At the same time, we must be aware that some older persons we encounter are so seriously ill that a return to normal, healthy functioning is not anticipated. Some suffer from irreversible conditions (Alzheimer's disease, metastasized cancer, advanced atherosclerosis) for which no cure is known. In such situations, improvement in the older person's physical condition is unlikely, and medical intervention is often aimed at slowing deterioration, alleviating pain, and helping the older person to function autonomously for as long as possible.

Situations such as this are often very frustrating for helping professionals. They are aware that regardless of their efforts, the medical prognosis is not likely to be reversed and that during their continuing association with their clients they will probably witness further deterioration. It is hard for them to conceptualize what a "successful" intervention might be. Unfortunately, this frustration leads many helping persons to wish to avoid the dying person. Because of their discomfort with death and because there appears to be little they can do to slow its course, some doctors, other health care workers, and social service workers limit the amount of time they spend with the dying. Families and friends, too, may disengage from the dying in efforts to ease the pain that eventual separation will cause or because they "don't know what to say to a dying person." Such abandonment is nearly always a mistake.

Probably the greatest fear of seriously impaired and dying persons is being left alone during their last months and days. It is important for helping persons to continue to provide support and assistance to such persons and their families. Sometimes help can be provided with concrete tasks (assistance in arranging for a will or a funeral, making the home, nursing home, or hospital environment more comfortable). For other persons the greatest need is to improve social relationships that take on importance in the face of death. In other cases, the dying person wants someone who is willing simply to talk or to maintain a quiet presence.

Helping professionals should take their cue from the dying person. One of the authors had a friend who died recently. During the last months of his life, one of this man's worries was his vegetable crop. When arrangements were made to harvest it, he was relieved that the issue was resolved. A minor point in the overall scheme of the universe, perhaps, but an important matter to a lifelong gardener, and important to our point that concrete help makes a difference. *Successful interventions are those aimed at listening carefully to the older person's wants and wishes and helping him or her realize them, providing resources to promote comfort, and providing support to family members who are caring for the dying person.* The worker's efforts are directed toward alleviating pain and helping the person to function as well as he or she can for as long as possible. Hospice programs do an excellent job of attempting to meet the needs of dying patients and their families, and adopt a philosophy of helping the dying person make the very best of the life yet to live. Persons who work with the aged should become well acquainted with hospice resources in their local communities and attempt to coordinate services on behalf of the dying older person.

Older Persons Are Our Future Selves

For many helping professionals working with older persons provokes considerable personal anxiety. This is because, barring an early death, we all know that we, too, will become old. As Abraham Monk (1977) points out, those who choose to work with unwed mothers, alcoholics, or renal dialysis patients "are attending to critical circumstances or conditions that they may never have to face in their own lives." Workers in aging, by contrast, are aware that they will likely become old and that their clients' problems of today may well be their own in the future. Young persons, far more than old ones, fear loss and death and will often go to great lengths to avoid contemplating the prospect of their own mortality.

We believe that one is unlikely to be effective in working with older persons unless one is willing to confront the inevitability of one's own aging and dying. Critical self-awareness is a key element in any effective human service practice, but it is particularly important for those attempting to work with the aged. One of the authors who frequently teaches aging courses to beginning students requires the students to contemplate their own aging at the outset of the course. Each student is asked to spend ten minutes in front of a mirror. The student is asked to think about how he or she will look at age seventy-five. Students are then asked to write an essay on this experience, incorporating their beliefs about what life will be like for them in advanced old age. Exercises such as this can be helpful in beginning to come to terms with one's own aging and mortality, but they can only scratch the surface. The ability to empathize with older persons with problems and to interact with them without anxiety develops with experience. It also requires that the professional engage in considerable hard work, examining personal goals and values and facing up to the fact that he or she will die sooner or later.

The notion that the aged are our future selves is also helpful to bear in mind as we interact with older persons and design interventions and new programs and policies to benefit them. We have already stressed the importance of respecting the older person's dignity and uniqueness. As we attempt to act according to this value, it may be helpful to think about how *we* would want to be treated as older recipients of service. Unfortunately, many helping persons communicate a lack of respect for their older clients through both verbal and nonverbal messages. It is important to show sensitivity by attention to the small details that tell people they are valued. Returning telephone calls instead of ignoring them, and showing up on time for appointments are two of these small things that can make big differences in how older people perceive themselves. One must remember that many older people have developed feelings of uselessness and mild depression because of the inconveniences to which they have been subjected by their social status, living conditions, or health problems. It is important not to add to this burden if one is to genuinely be of help.

The authors have known helping professionals (often decades younger than their clients) who automatically assume that it is appropriate to address older persons by their first names. While a few older persons are comfortable with this practice, most are not. It communicates a lack of respect for their years of experience and tends to reinforce whatever negative feelings of dependency they may already have developed. It also gives the impression that they are being viewed as children. We strongly advise you to address older people by the formal title they prefer (Mr., Mrs., Miss, Ms., Dr., Col., and so on) unless they explicitly ask you to do otherwise.

As a sidelight, we must point out that to a certain generation of women, the "Miss" is as important as "Ms." may be to many younger women. We know never-married older women who wear the title "Miss" like a badge of honor because it expresses their independence in a way that is meaningful to them. One should not force them to accept new symbols if they wish to retain the old.

Another instance of communicating lack of respect is speaking of persons as if they were their disorders. We are all familiar with hospital personnel who refer to "the ulcer in 204" and "the coronary in 406." While there may be a need to classify the problems of older persons for record-keeping purposes, it does not follow that their whole lives should be subsumed under the name of a disease. How one is identified is important. Referring to a female as a "broad" is quite different than referring to her as a "woman." Symbols are important to people, and this is as it should be. Few people, regardless of their age, relish the idea of being thought of as a disease. Those who work with older persons should be aware of the inherent danger in using labels to describe older persons and should be careful not to depersonalize in this way.

An additional notion to bear in mind is that older persons, just like younger ones, want to participate actively in decisions made about their lives. The principle of self-determination is important in our culture in general and in the helping professions in particular. Basically it means that people should have the right to decide for themselves, unless what they decide is clearly harmful or unhealthy, either for themselves or for others. This principle is, however, often overlooked in dealings with older persons, particularly if they are ill or dependent. Workers and families have been known to collaborate and make decisions in the older person's "best interest," without having consulted the intended beneficiary at all. Such denial of the right to self-determination can have devastating effects, particularly when the decision involves major life changes. On the basis of long experience in helping residents adjust to nursing homes, Elaine Brody (1977) argues that older persons should participate to the fullest extent possible in the decision to seek nursing home care and the decision about which nursing home to enter. When older people have some say in the decision to relocate and participate in the selection process, they are far more likely to adjust successfully than when they do not.

The notions of choice and self-determination are of particular importance for the very dependent aged. For such persons, the ranges within which life choices can be made are often extremely limited, particularly if these persons reside in an institutional setting. Thus, trivial as it may appear, giving people choices about which of three desserts they would like served to them at lunch or about what time of day they would prefer to have their bath can be extremely important. The freedom to make such choices helps seriously impaired older persons retain a degree of autonomy and independence and serves to protect their dignity as adults.

Thinking of today's older persons as "our future selves" can also help us sort through our values about how current societal arrangements could be altered to make for the most conducive environment for our own old age. Ageist policies and practices that are instituted and perpetuated when we are younger may well affect us in our own old age. Can we, for example, favor urban planning schemes that isolate those unable to drive automobiles when we know that we, too, may be unable to drive in advanced old age? Do we support efforts to move older workers out of the labor force when we know that such policies may limit our own work opportunities later in life? Would *we* feel comfortable receiving services from the agencies and facilities that currently serve older persons in our communities? Our answers to these and other similar questions should influence our efforts to combat ageist practices where we see them and our activities as advocates for the rights of older persons. When we treat the older persons we encounter today with dignity and respect and when we develop policies, programs, and organizations that take into account older persons' wants and their freedom of choice, we are not only improving the quality of life for today's aged, but we are also working toward a better environment for our own old age.

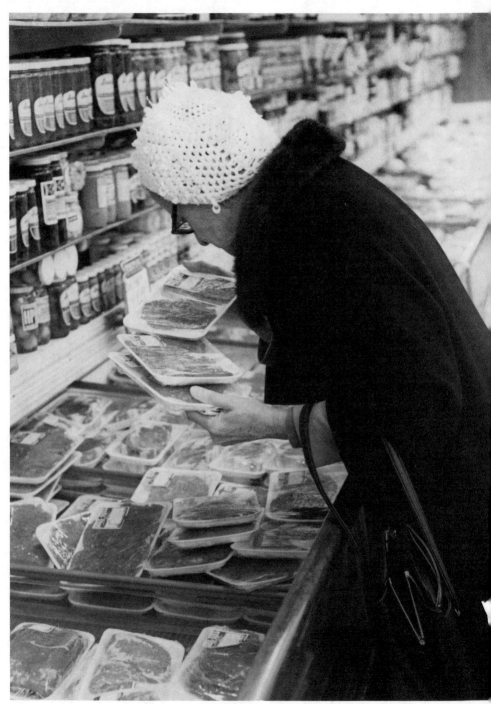

3

Economic Resources

In this chapter, we will focus on the resources available to satisfy the economic wants of older persons. Because this is a book about services to older persons, we will devote most of the space to those economic resources about which service personnel need to know in order to provide appropriate counsel to the elderly.

As we are all aware, everyone needs some dependable source of money in order to purchase the goods and services necessary to maintain life. Ordinarily, this means income from a job, business, or profession. This familiar activity is used by some older people, but many either choose to retire, are retired as a consequence of company or institutional policy, or retire due to poor health. Others, who were poor and marginally employed when they were younger, remain poor when they are old. Obviously, the economic resources that one commands are intimately related to whether one will age successfully. In a money economy, those with inadequate resources will have a harder time of it than those who have enough.

As we saw in chapter 1, the poverty rate among persons sixty-five and over is lower than the rate in the general population. It was shown that older persons in general have a higher net worth than was the case historically. However, this cheerful news should not obscure the conditions of those who have not shared in the general affluence of the post World War II period.

It is our conviction that in an ideal world the economic system ought to operate in a way that permits everyone to have a decent level of living. Few would argue with this ideal. The difficulties arise around two questions: (1) How does one ensure a decent level of living for everyone? and (2) How much is enough?

Providing a Decent Level of Living ─────────

While we do not intend to get into an extended discussion of economic theory, some brief comments may be helpful at this point. There are three basic (and mutually exclusive) answers to the first question.

1. The best way to ensure the highest level of economic prosperity for the greatest number of people is through an economic system in which prices, wages, and wealth are determined by the workings of the market. The market should, ideally, operate with as little governmental influence as possible.
2. The best way to ensure the highest level of economic prosperity for the greatest number of people is through a system in which the central government acts as trustee for the people and controls the distribution of income, wealth, and social privileges.
3. The best way to ensure the highest level of economic prosperity for the greatest number of people is through a system in which markets operate under some level of government supervision and restraint. The role of the government is to smooth out the rough workings of the market through the regulation of both fiscal and monetary policy. Regulating fiscal policy involves adjusting the rate and amount of governmental taxation and spending. Monetary policy refers to those activities of the government that affect the creation of money and credit.

There are no operating examples of a pure market economy. In the latter half of the nineteenth century, Britain and the United States approximated the pure market economy more nearly than any other modern nations. The socialist economies of Eastern Europe and Asia are examples of the second alternative, although, increasingly, they are adopting market elements.

Most Western nations and a number of Asian countries, most notably Japan, and Korea, are "mixed" economies of the third type. In those countries, both market forces and governmental regulation complement each other in providing the economic resources that support a relatively higher standard of living for more people than the socialist economies have been able to do. The mix of governmental activity and market activity varies in these nations from Austria, where the government is clearly the major player, to the United States, where the market is predominant.

Therefore, in practical terms, our society attempts to answer the question of how to ensure a decent level of living by a combination of private support, market-related activities, and governmental programs to smooth out the roughest spots. Presently, we will look at these elements as they affect older Americans.

How Much Is Enough?

This is not an easy question. How much is enough for you? Couldn't you use more money if you had it? A bigger house or apartment? Newer appliances and more comfortable furniture? Longer and more luxurious vacations? Of course you could! There is no upper limit to what one might want when he or she thinks about it.

However, there is a practical limit. One develops a certain style of living over the course of his or her life. This style of living is related to a variety of things—personal taste, geographical and cultural traditions, and the amount of money available for use. This latter point is most important. Clearly, those persons with the most income and wealth have a wider range of choices. Those with limited resources throughout the life course develop a narrower range of preferences as a result of more restricted choices. Are wealth and privilege fairly distributed? That is, are wealth and privilege distributed in a way that most people would see as deserved according to some generally accepted standard? No. When it comes to the distribution of economic goods and services, no society has completely solved the problem of equity. There is always some imbalance and some people have resources that others do not think are deserved while some lack resources that, in a fair world, they probably should have. *None of the three alternative means of organizing economic systems—market, governmentally managed, or mixed—completely answers the question of economic fairness.*

In the Direction of Equity

We *can* say that we believe in equity (or "fairness") as an ideal. As we discuss resources, we will tend to value most those things that seem to us to be as nearly fair as is possible in the real world. Fairness does not demand economic equality. People who have done well economically (provided that they have done well honestly, of course) should be able to benefit from their hard work, ability, and luck. We are not going to recommend that the assets of one class should be confiscated to benefit another. However, we do think that there should be a decent standard of living that should be attainable through some combination of market and governmental activity.

What Is a "Decent Standard"?

Some years ago, the federal government adopted the approach that is used to determine the poverty line. Based on a 1955 survey by the U.S. Department of Agriculture that suggested that families spent one-third of their after-tax income on food, a minimally adequate diet was designed, and its market cost was multiplied by three. This figure, adjusted for family size, became the official poverty line. Each year, this figure is adjusted to take into account the increase in the Consumer Price Index. In chapter 1, we reported that in 1985, the poverty line for one person was $5,156 while for two it was $6,503. These official figures, we pointed out, do not take into account the value of medical care, food stamps, or federal participation in housing. With those taken into account, the level of poverty among those aged sixty-five and over declines to around 3 percent.

A major problem with the official poverty line, however, is that there are "hidden" poor who do not get included. The poor persons who live with relatives may not officially have fewer resources, but in practice they may not have a claim on enough family resources to escape real poverty.

While it is encouraging to find that absolute poverty has been drastically reduced among the elderly, simply being nonpoor does not mean that one has enough to age successfully.

We live in Alabama where incomes and prices are below the national average. Using figures that are conveniently at hand, we have calculated the following rough estimate of what we would consider a decent standard of living for a couple aged sixty-five or over living in a small- or moderate-sized city in Alabama.

Proposed Monthly Budget for a Couple Aged 65 or Over
(based on 1985 prices)

Food	$250.00	(roughly a USDA "moderate" diet)
Housing	250.00	(this will rent a two-bedroom apartment in a small or moderate-sized city)
Utilities	90.00	(750 KWH electricity, 50 cu. ft. gas)
Clothing	50.00	(modest replacement costs)
Telephone	25.00	(this does not allow for many long distance calls of a long duration)
Auto	22.00	(100 miles at $.22 per mile)
Water	15.00	(includes garbage pickup)
Medicare	50.00	(Part B, see Chapter 4)
Other	60.00	(recreation, dental bills, incidentals)
	$812.00	

Annualized, this would mean about $9,800 per year per couple. This amount would provide a decent standard of living for an older couple living in a small town or city in Alabama. Another $900 per year, bringing the total to a little over $10,600, would allow a modest amount of leeway to handle insurance, some savings for replacement or repair of an automobile, and the purchase of items that add to human comfort. Since about 80 percent of Americans sixty-five or over own their own homes, and since most of these have paid-up mortgages, the amount projected for housing could be used for repairs and upkeep. This is not luxury living, but a very modest estimate of at least a decent level of living. This amount of money would not be enough in more expensive parts of the country. However, it should be possible to adjust this standard, depending on local costs. Of course, this does not take into account catastrophic illness or a major purchase—a new car, for example—but simply a very moderate standard, a target amount that would enable a couple to live in some dignity.

This figure is about one-and-a-half times the current poverty line. It is unlikely that Americans would accept abandoning the notion of a poverty line in favor of a "moderate comfort" line for all age groups. It is also unlikely that such a scheme would be acceptable even if it only applied to those sixty-five and over. Raising all persons sixty-five and over to this standard (when adjusted for local differences) through public funds would be very expensive, and Americans are not currently in the mood to tax themselves further for this purpose. However, we think that it is useful to have a target income against which to judge adequacy in a given area.

For some years before 1982, when their own budget cuts caused them to stop, the Bureau of Labor Statistics (BLS) produced a series of annual Retired Couple's Budgets. For 1981, they set the intermediate level at $10,226 (Schulz, 1985:39). Our tentative budget is comparable, since inflation has been relatively low since 1981. It also compares fairly well even though the BLS budget was national in scope and ours was based on a small- or medium-sized southern city where costs are lower.

Now let us turn to the question of how older Americans actually contend with "the wolf at the door," as poverty was classically described.

In chapter 1 we noted that the mean household income for persons sixty-five and over was $18,279. For whites it was $18,790, for blacks it was $12,042, and for persons of Spanish origin it was $14,045. These figures clearly remove the average older American from poverty. The trouble is that averages obscure individuals. Actually, 12 percent of Americans sixty-five and over have household incomes of less than

$5,000 per year and another 26 percent have incomes between $5,000 and $10,000 per year (*Statistical Abstract 1987*, p.432). While there may be other resources that prevent these people from actually sinking under the poverty line, it is clear that nearly one-third of Americans sixty-five and over do not have enough current income to suggest that they live with the degree of economic security that we think represents genuinely successful aging.

Sources of Income for the Aged

There are several sources of income for older Americans. We will examine the major ones here.

Employment

Approximately three million persons aged sixty-five and over (about 10.5 percent of all persons sixty-five and over) are counted in what the Census Bureau terms the *civilian labor force*. About 1.8 million are men and 1.2 million are women. Together, these men and women make up about 3 percent of the labor force. Of those considered part of the work force, about 97 percent are actually employed. About 97 percent of white males in this category are employed as are about 91 percent of male members of minority groups. The employment rate of white females and females who are members of a minority group is almost equal (96 percent and 95 percent, respectively). Of course, as the reader may know, there may actually be more older persons who would like to work, but have been dropped from the official work force by failing to be counted among those actively seeking work. And, quite obviously, about 90 percent of persons sixty-five and over are not considered in the work force to begin with. Further, some of those who are counted as employed are employed only part time.

Of those persons sixty-five and over who are employed, approximately 55 percent of the men and 48 percent of the women are paid wages with median hourly rates of $5.16 for men and $4.51 for women. The discrepancy between women's versus men's wages thus continues in the older ranges of the work force.

Clearly, then, employment is not a major factor in providing persons sixty-five and over with an adequate standard of living. While work, either at hourly rates or in a business or profession, is an option for some, it is not a solution for 90 percent of older Americans. Since most older Americans are not poor, this is not a crucial problem. As a matter of fact, the number of older Americans who work has declined. Ycas and Grad (1987) report that in a 1962 study, 36 percent of those sixty-five or over had earnings from work, while by 1984, the percentage had fallen to 21. However, there is still a small minority of healthy older Americans who may want and need to work. Professionals should recognize that work may be a realistic idea for a number of older persons. As mentioned in chapter 1, some businesses are willing to hire older workers, at least on a part-time basis. Therefore, it will be helpful if the professional knows of opportunities for work to which older workers can be referred.

Social Security

Over 90 percent of Americans sixty-five and over receive benefits from Old Age, Survivors, Disability, and Health Insurance (OASDHI), commonly known as Social Security. (Actually, the Social Security Act includes a number of provisions, known as titles, but most people use the term Social Security to mean OASDHI.) Since over 95 percent of American workers are now covered, the percentage of persons receiving benefits will increase. For 62 percent of those who receive benefits, OASDHI is the source of half or more of their income (Ycas and Grad, 1987). In 1987, the average monthly benefit for a retired worker was $492. A 4.2 percent cost-of-living increase brought the average benefit up to $513 for 1988. In the case of a married couple, the average benefit rose to $770 per month. The size of one's benefit depends roughly on the amount of money that one earned during his or her working years, assuming that one has earned at least forty calendar quarters of covered employment. The formula by which benefits are calculated is complicated (see "Social Security in Review," an unsigned regular feature, in the *Social Security Bulletin*, January 1988). The formula is deliberately constructed to favor the lower income beneficiary. The benefits are not open-ended. The maximum benefit for a single person was about $800 in 1987, while a couple with maximum benefits would have gotten about $1,200 per month, regardless of how much money they earned during their working years. Since most older Americans receive benefits from the system, we will go into some detail about how it operates.

OASDHI was created by the Social Security Act of 1935. It was part of President Franklin D. Roosevelt's New Deal, which was a series of federal programs designed to mitigate the impact of the Great Depression of the 1930s. Social Security is basically a pay-as-you-go system.

The basic idea is that today's workers and their employers pay a special tax on salaries. Self-employed people pay a tax on the proceeds from their professions or businesses that is approximately equal to the tax paid by both the employee and the employer. These taxes go into three "trust funds." There is one fund for Old Age and Survivors' Insurance, a second one for Disability Insurance, and a third for Health Insurance. There is a fourth fund, but this is for the accumulation of Part B Medicare funds, part of which come from optional monthly premiums paid by the beneficiary (see chapter 4). Money taken from the trust funds pays the benefits to those persons currently eligible. The trust funds exist mainly for accounting purposes.

While OASDHI is often described as social insurance, it really is a tax designed to redistribute income from those who are working to those who have retired, become permanently and totally disabled, or are the dependents of deceased or disabled wage earners. The program was called social insurance in order to make it more palatable to the voters of the 1930s. People understood how insurance worked. They could understand the idea of a trust fund and the notion that one was paying into a system that would provide some income in old age. The notion of an intergenerational income transfer had no meaning to the voters of the 1930s and doesn't mean very much to the average person now.

Actually, these are not trust funds in the sense in which this term is generally used. In a genuine trust fund, the money is invested as a separate identifiable account that is managed for the good of the beneficiary. The money is "there," and the institution managing the trust must be able to account for it.

In the case of the Social Security System, the money is taxed from this generation's workers and passes through the trust funds in payments to beneficiaries. One's Social Security account is, therefore, not an account in that one has a bank account. Rather, it is a promise on the part of the government to pay benefits. Ordinarily the trust fund contains only enough money to pay the current year's benefits. Beginning in 1983, however, a surplus has been accumulating so that there will be enough money to meet the needs of the baby boomers.

When one retires (at sixty-five for full benefit or at sixty-two if one is willing to take a reduced benefit), his or her initial benefit payment is calculated. Benefit increase is tied to the increase in the Consumer Price Index or the increase in wages for urban wage earners and clerical workers, whichever is the lower.

Originally, increases in benefits were decided annually by Congress. In 1972, Congress tied benefits to increases in the federal cost of living index. This resulted in a benefit structure that rapidly outstripped the tax income. Since the cost of living was rising faster than incomes, the net result would have been to pay retired workers a larger benefit than their actual salaries had been. These overindexed benefits became known as windfall benefits. When Congress realized that they had seriously overindexed the benefits, they corrected the imbalance starting with the benefits of 1977. While they did not decrease any benefits, they did reduce the rate at which they were scheduled to increase. Persons born between 1917 and 1921 did not get the windfall benefits, because they were born during what came to be called the notch between the time the government started to adjust the benefits and the time when the adjustment was completed. Some "notch babies" have become very angry at the system and have lobbied to have the excess benefits restored, but the system has resolutely argued that these benefits were not intended in the first place, and therefore the notch babies are not entitled to them. Persons who work with older Americans may encounter a number of notch babies and will do well to avoid becoming involved in a very emotional argument. Explanations have been made by the Social Security system, but many notch babies are still extremely upset about the situation.

Originally, the system was aimed at industrial workers. In 1940, before the first benefits were paid, benefits were added for dependents (wives, children, widowed mothers, or dependent parents of a deceased worker). The program, which started as Old Age Insurance (OAI) became Old Age and Survivors' Insurance (OASI). In the 1950s, benefits for disabled workers and their dependents were added and the program became Old Age, Survivors' and Disability Insurance (OASDI). In the 1960s, benefits were added to enable older persons to pay some of their hospital and doctor bills (Medicare). Thus, the system became Old Age, Survivors', Disability, and Health Insurance (OASDHI). Over the years, more and more workers (including farm workers, domestic workers, and even persons in religious orders) have been brought into the system. In the late 1930s, each worker paid a tax of 2 percent of the first $1,500 in wages and his or her employer paid a similar amount. Thus, each worker paid a maximum tax of $30 a year that was matched by his or her employer. As of 1988, the payroll tax is 7.51 percent on the first $45,000 of income, matched by the employer. The self-employed will pay 13.02 percent of their first $45,000. Over the years, the tax rate and the salary that is subject to the tax have increased. As of this writing, the maximum tax is scheduled to top out at 7.65 percent by 1990. The amount of income subject to the tax is dependent on the economy using a formula devised for the purpose.

Most self-employed people were included in the system during the 1950s. Self-employed people initially paid a tax rate that was about half again as much as the rate paid by wage earners. Gradually, the tax on self-employed people has risen. It is currently scheduled to reach 15.3 percent in 1990.

One of the unsolved problems in the system relates to the taxation of married women's benefits and the subsequent influence of that tax on what they get out of the system. In order to get the maximum payment, the system calculates the basic benefit on the larger of the two salaries earned by the couple. The spouse benefit is then half that amount. Given the past history of discrimination toward women in the work force, the larger salary is usually that of the husband. The woman is usually better off if she takes half of the husband's benefit. Consider this example. A husband earns $20,000 per year while his wife earns $10,000. At retirement, the wife has two choices. She can take a benefit based on her salary, or she can take half her husband's benefit. She will maximize the family's benefit by taking half her husband's benefit, since it would be larger than her individual benefit. However, she would get half of her husband's benefit even if she had never worked outside the home. What benefit accrues from the Social Security taxes that she has paid? About the only consolation that the spouse who earns the lesser income can have is in remembering that Social Security "contributions" are a transfer tax that provided income to the previous generation.

Of course, if the wife had the larger income, it would be the husband who would not directly benefit from the taxes that he paid, but this is not the usual case.

The current system is based on family norms of the 1930s (that is, husband as wage earner, wife as homemaker). It has not been revised to recognize that most wives now work outside the home. Various reform proposals have been advanced, but they have been shelved because of the cost involved.

At this time, over 95 percent of those who earn income in the United States are subject to the tax and eligible for benefits. Very few groups are excluded, and those who are are special cases. An example is state university professors in Illinois. They chose to be excluded before such exclusion was prohibited. In most other states, professors are included.

A series of free pamphlets is available at your local Social Security office. It would be a good idea to pick some of them up in order to have up-to-date information. Two are especially helpful: *History of Social Security*, and *Your Social Security*. The former contains a table showing the benefit increases since 1939, the changes in the earnings base and tax rates over the years, and an outline of the changes in coverage. The latter contains a great deal of information on the system's benefits and how to apply for them. Each pamphlet is updated periodically.

We mentioned earlier that there was a lot of misinformation about the system. Let us look at a few things we have read or heard and offer an explanation that may be helpful to the reader. While it is probably useless to become involved in arguments about the following issues, it is still better to know the facts. It may prevent the service professional from becoming embroiled in useless controversy.

1. "The Social Security System is going broke! There won't be any money when I retire!" Periodically, the popular press prints articles whose titles are more sensational than the text. We have two in our files: "How Secure Is Your Social Security?" by Bernard Gavzer (Gavzer, 1987) and "Can Social Security Be Saved?" by Peter G. Peterson (Peterson, 1983). People see articles of this sort and become inordinately concerned about them. The truth is that the Social Security System will pay benefits as long as the Congress of the United States is subject to election and persons sixty-five and over have votes! When problems have appeared in the system, Congress has acted to solve them. While it is true that the problems have often been of Congress' own making (the overindexing of benefits in 1977, for example), the fact that senators and representatives are political animals ensures that the system's commitments will be honored. The system will probably undergo changes, but it has paid benefits for nearly fifty years and appears to be solvent on its current basis well into the next century.

2. "I paid in the money and I am entitled to it!" Actually, beneficiaries get a lot more money than they paid in. In Gavzer's article cited above, he describes his own situation. He got his Social Security card in 1941. He has paid $20,490.63 in taxes. If he retired at age sixty-seven, he would get $9,480 a year, based on the formula that determines benefits. If he lives to age seventy-nine, he will get at least $142,200—even if there are no increases in benefits.

The benefits, then, are not really tied to "contributions" in the sense that income from an annuity would be. If one bought an annuity from an insurance company, his or her benefits would be very clearly related to his or her investment. The money used to purchase the annuity goes into an account on the company's books and is a clearly identifiable obligation of the company. In Social Security, one's benefits are related to the will of Congress. The tax that today's retired worker paid went to earlier beneficiaries. The tax that you pay goes into the trust funds and out to your parents or grandparents. How much they get depends on Congress' willingness to tax and your willingness to be taxed!

3. "The president wants to cut my check!" Since Congress has, on occasion, raised benefits generously, they have outrun revenues. The usual response has been to broaden the tax base by adding more work-

ers to the system, increasing the taxes, and raising the amount of income subject to the tax. Since over 95 percent of American workers are now covered, there are few unincluded occupational groups that can be brought into the system. Future increases, barring any major change in the way the system operates, will mean either higher tax rates or the inclusion of more income in the tax base. When the benefits outrun the contributions, somebody has to consider doing something about it. One possibility is to limit the increase in benefits; no one's check is cut. What happens is that next year's increase isn't as big. This has happened in 1977 and again in 1983 when the formula for benefit increase was changed.

Since OASDHI is a retirement program, there are limits to how much one can earn through employment in a given period until one reaches age seventy. This amount changes annually. Retired persons under sixty-five can now (as of 1988) earn up to $6,120 before facing a reduction in benefits. Persons aged sixty-five to sixty-nine can earn $8,400. One's benefit is reduced $1 for every $2 earned over these income limits. This is not an overall cut in the benefits of the system, but a standard provision that has been in effect for some time.

Service professionals who work with older persons may hear these and other feelings expressed. Argument will probably be pointless. The best solution would be to either refer the individual to the local Social Security office or to ask someone from that office to come to a group meeting of older persons. Persons who work for Social Security are prepared to deal with these questions.

Social Security and Income Adequacy ———

If a couple received the average benefit of about $770 a month, they would probably be able to get by if they had a small amount of additional income and lived in the rural South. Indeed, the lower cost of living has drawn many older people to that area. However, not everybody wants to live in a small Southern town, even though it does have much to recommend it! Further, recall that this would be a moderate standard of living and does not include enough for any really serious emergency. Fortunately, most older people have income in addition to Social Security. For those who do not have additional sources of income, emergencies are often catastrophic.

Social Security wasn't designed to be the whole source of support for the retired worker. In its publications, the Social Security System has repeatedly stressed that OASDI payments are intended to be "one leg of a three-legged stool." The other two legs are savings and pension benefits from one's employer. The Social Security System's publications often put it this way: Social Security should be regarded as a basic economic floor upon which one is supposed to build one's retirement income. The difficulty, of course, is that some people do not work for one employer long enough to earn significant pension benefits, and persons with low incomes seldom are able to save a significant amount of money.

Private Pensions and Savings

Many persons earn pension benefits from employment. Some may also have their own personalized pension plan built around some savings plan or the income from assets.

Assets in some form have become important. Ycas and Grad (1987) report that "the proportion with at least some asset income rose from 54 percent to 68 percent between 1962 and 1984, and the share of aggregate income from assets increased from 16 percent to 28 percent, second only to Social Security payments" (p. 7). Of course, income-producing assets are more likely to be held by those who had higher incomes before retirement.

About 8.5 percent of the household units comprised of Americans aged sixty-five and over have invested in Individual Retirement Accounts (IRAs) or the so-called Keogh plans. Before the tax reforms of 1987, all workers could put up to $2,000 per year into an IRA and deduct the amount deposited from their gross annual income. Unemployed spouses were permitted to deposit $250 per year in these accounts. Since the tax reform, these deductions are no longer allowed if one has any other tax-deferred savings plan and has a net taxable income of $45,000 or more. The interest earned is still tax deferred until the owner of the account begins to draw money from it. The Keogh plan is a similar kind of tax-deferral plan for self-employed people. A number of retirees will have money in these accounts, but since the IRA is a relatively new investment plan, it probably will not affect a large number of older persons in the near future. The median value of these accounts in 1984 (the last year for which figures were available at this writing) was $6,369. Since the sale of IRAs and Keogh plans has been heavier in younger age groups, their impact on the income of persons sixty-five and over will be more substantial in later years. For low-income workers who do not have any other tax-deferred pension plan, the IRA is a good idea, but it obviously depends upon one's ability to save.

For many formerly employed persons, the company pension is a major source of retirement income. Some $90 billion are invested in private pension plans and another $65 billion in pension plans at various levels of government. Ycas and Grad (1987) note that "almost three times as many aged couples and single persons received employer pensions in 1984 as in 1962—24 percent of the aged had pensions from private former employers and 14 percent had pensions earned as former employees of federal, state, or local governments" (p. 7). While government employees' pension systems are generally dependable, there are problems with pensions from private industry. Although most private pension plans are subject to the safeguards of the Employment Retirement Income Security Act of 1974 (see Schulz, 1985, p. 160), problems remain. For example, one usually has to work for a company for a number of years (ten to thirty) in order to acquire a vested interest in the plan. When one has a vested interest, his or her pension benefits are guaranteed. Workers who changed jobs frequently may not earn significant coverage, and the benefits for unvested workers are usually not portable to other employers. Consequently, older persons with unstable work records may not receive anything from company pensions. A further problem is that many plans may be underfunded and may not be able to pay the benefits, especially if the company goes out of business.

While it is hard to generalize about the amount of income a person will likely receive, it is obvious that persons with good salaries or wages who have worked for a long time for one company will do better at pension time than will persons with lower salaries and less seniority.

Supplemental Security Income

The Social Security Act of 1935 incorporated a provision for a need-based welfare payment for persons sixty-five and older in the title on Public Assistance. Before the act, a number of states had adopted "pension" plans for older residents. These pensions, which were not pensions at all, but public assistance grants, were financed entirely from state and local funds. Generally, they were very small and were far from adequate.

As is the case with other parts of the Public Assistance provisions of the Social Security Act, states were given the option to design a state program for means-tested assistance payments for older people. A means test requires the applicant to prove need, based on a standard definition. Soon all states developed state plans, as was required in order to qualify for federal matching funds. The act required that each state develop a criterion by which need was judged and appropriate money to pay its share of the grants "up front." The federal government then matched the state's appropriation according to a formula. Effectively, the federal government contributed about one-half of the grant. Because these grants were developed at the state level, they were conditioned upon the state's willingness to tax its citizens for the purpose.

The result was that there was great variety in the size of the grants among the states. In 1974, three public assistance programs (Old Age Assistance, Aid to the Blind, and Aid to the Permanently and Totally Disabled) were combined into what is now known as Supplemental Security Income (SSI). The combined programs are now administered by the Social Security system using the same offices as OASDHI personnel. With the shift from state to federal operation, national minimum benefits and eligibility standards were adopted, eliminating some of the variation. States can, and many do, supplement the federal grants; therefore, variation persists. There still is a means test.

Payments currently average about $180 per month per person. There are many poor older persons who receive both an OASDHI payment and an SSI payment. This happens when the person's OASDHI and personal resources are not enough to lift him or her above the poverty level. In these cases, the SSI payment is, in fact, a supplement to other income. This is why the average grant is relatively low. For those with no OASDHI or other income, the grant from SSI will be larger than the average. As of this writing, an individual who lives in a state with no supplement and who has no other income could receive $354 per month from SSI. A couple would get $532.

Food Stamps

Historically, there has been a controversy about in-kind versus cash relief of poverty. In-kind relief includes any form of noncash relief—food, clothing, housing, or other direct grant of goods to the poor. Over the centuries, the pendulum has swung back and forth between these two forms of relief. Today, most authorities support the giving of direct cash grants, allowing the consumer to purchase his or her wants. However, there are still some aspects of the complex American welfare system that reflect the beliefs of an earlier day.

Rent vouchers are one such remnant. Food stamps are another. In the 1930s, one of the government's attempts to support farm production involved buying up surplus farm produce. Some of this surplus was stored against potential future shortages. The problem was that shortages did not occur. Besides, some of the produce didn't lend itself to storage. As the storage program got too expensive—and after some products spoiled, an event that usually received wide press coverage—the federal government conceived of the notion of giving the produce away. Many recipients of Old Age Assistance qualified for receipt of the surplus commodities.

Persons meeting a means test would queue up at the county's distribution centers on the first of the month. They would be given a carton of food. While the contents varied, depending on what produce was currently in surplus, the carton usually contained a large tin of chopped ham, a sack of flour, a bag of sugar, corn meal, powdered eggs, some dried beans or peas, a pound of butter, and a box of powdered milk. One of the authors recalls being invited to a county welfare office for lunch where the food was prepared from the contents of a box of commodities as a demonstration of the high quality of the food. The meal was quite decent, but high in starch.

As the federal government changed its policies and made subsidy payments to encourage farmers to hold land out of production instead of buying up of commodities, the distribution was curtailed. Today, surplus commodities are generally limited to butter and cheese, since other produce is usually not purchased as an economic support measure.

As a curious sidelight on the distribution of commodities, one of the authors once was driving by a distribution point and saw one of his golfing partners—a man with quite sufficient income—standing in the butter and cheese line. He was poorly dressed—his taste in clothing is suspect anyway—and he was preparing to represent himself as eligible. At that time, there was inevitably some confusion about identifying those who were eligible. The author stopped his car and tried to harass the potential recipient into giving up his fraud, but the effort was unsuccessful. The man was seen later carrying his pound of butter and two pounds of cheese. This example is not intended to make light of a serious problem, but to point out that the commodities program was subject to abuse from clever and plausible people.

In place of the commodity distribution, we now have the federal food stamp program. To be eligible, a household can have no more than $1,500 in assets (a house and one car are exempted) and a gross income below 130 percent of the current poverty level. In effect, food stamps are available only to those who can demonstrate poverty; they are not a general resource for the average older person.

There have been abuses in the food stamp program, just as was possible when commodities were distributed. Counterfeit stamps have been recovered by the police. There has also been a brisk trade in the stamps, as recipients traded them for things other than food (they may not be used to purchase nonfood items at the store). Generally, however, the control of the program is tighter than it initially was, and most food stamps appear to be used as they were intended. Persons working with poor older people should be sure that their clients or patients know of the program and should refer the older person to the county welfare office for determination of eligibility.

Low-Cost Community Services

In most communities, there are various money-saving devices available to older persons. Generally, there is no means test for these things. Many drugstores give senior citizen discounts for prescriptions. Moving picture theaters may offer reduced admission prices. There may be discounts on public transportation.

In most larger communities, there will be subsidized housing for older people, but there will usually be a means test. Some communities also have energy assistance plans that range from deferred payment plans for heat and light bills to actual home repairs that decrease heating costs. These, too, will most likely require a means test.

In addition to the above, there may be other places where older persons may be able to save money, but they are not well known. The mental health clinic may have a reduced fee for low-income people. Some civic organizations may have special facilities or resources that are available to older persons.

Professionals who work with older persons should become familiar with the variety of ways in which older persons can augment their basic resources by using these cost-cutting services in the community.

Tax Benefits

Persons sixty-five and over each receive two personal deductions instead of one on their federal income tax. This is fairly well known. Less well known is that all states provide property tax relief for older persons. In some states, there is what is called a homestead exemption, which provides for an exemption from property taxes on a home that one owns. Generally, the homestead exemption applies to all older persons, regardless of their financial status. Other states provide a tax reduction based on financial need.

Payments from Relatives

Of course, some older people may receive regular money payments from their children or other relatives. In a recent study, the Census Bureau estimated that about 15 percent of those persons receiving help from relatives are older family members. The average amount of these payments was about $1,400 per year (*Birmingham News-Birmingham Post-Herald*, Oct. 29, 1988, p. A 10). While it is commendable that relatives help, the problem is simply that such help is undependable and, at best, can only be considered a conditional resource for older people.

The Future

Ycas and Grad (1987) report on a survey of new beneficiaries of Social Security. The picture presented is quite positive. Newly retired persons are better off than those who retired earlier. Many were still working (27 percent of the single retirees and 44 percent of the couples), and the subjects tended to be relatively young. Eighty-four percent of the couples (73 percent of the single women and 63 percent of the single men) had income from assets—mainly interest from savings accounts, although most did not have more than $100 in income from assets. About half of the retired workers had pensions from public or private employers. Single women were more likely to have pensions than single men, but their pensions were about $150 a month lower. A few of the men (8 to 10 percent) got veterans' benefits. Only 2 percent of the married couples and 7 percent of the unmarried received SSI payments. Only 3 percent of married couples and 11 percent of the single retirees were entirely dependent upon Social Security for 100 percent of their income.

We can do no better than to quote Ycas and Grad about the future prospects for the financial health of the aged: "Despite the increase in life expectancy and the decline in the labor-force participation among the elderly, . . . there is good reason to hope that the financial position of the aged population in the United States will continue to improve for some years to come" (p. 14).

4

Physical Health

Without question, one of the most important components in successful aging is satisfactory physical health. Older persons without health restrictions have the opportunity to take part in a far wider range of potentially fulfilling activities than do their peers with health problems. As is discussed in Chapter 6, people in good health have a wider range of suitable housing choices than do those whose health is poor. And because being in poor health can be expensive—even for older persons eligible for Medicare—those in good health can use more of their income on enjoyable activities. It is not surprising that study after study has found that one of the most important predictors of "satisfaction with life" in old age has been good health (Larson, 1978).

Good physical health is critical to successful aging. Thus, professionals who serve the old focus a great deal of their attention on providing programs and services that promote good health and that help older persons who have health problems to cope more satisfactorily with them. Since physical health problems are common in old age, it is very important that professionals who work with the aged have a basic understanding of them, the limitations that these problems place on daily living, and the resources that are available.

First we discuss the general health status of the older population and the types of deviations from good health that are most common among older persons. We focus on how health problems can be prevented, how they are treated once they occur, and what the implications (both of the health condition and its treatment) are for successful social functioning. We also consider the resources that are available to older persons to promote healthful living. This discussion focuses on the types of professionals and facilities the older person might use in seeking optimum health. We also discuss financial resources that are available to help the older person pay for health care services. The ultimate objective is to help the human service professional assist older persons to attain a satisfying level of physical health or, if this is not possible, to cope as well as they can with limitations that cannot be corrected.

A Definition of
Satisfactory Physical Health

Satisfaction with a person's health is a relative concept. The World Health Organization (1946), for example, defines health as a "state of complete physical, mental, and social well-being, not merely the absence of disease or infirmity." This definition suggests an ideal that few of us (young or old) are likely to meet all of the time.

Another standard we can use to assess satisfactory health is the judgment of physicians and other health professionals. Having examined a person, a physician makes an assessment of a person's health status, noting negative conditions that can be corrected, those that cannot be corrected but can be alleviated, and those that are unlikely to respond to any known treatments. Physicians are likely to be unsatisfied with a person's health until a reversible dysfunctional condition has been corrected. They are also likely to rate a person's health as unsatisfactory when a persistent problem cannot be treated. It should be noted, however, that physicians and other health professionals also assess health in a relative way. A problem that may be labeled unsatisfactory in a twenty year old (for example, moderately elevated blood pressure) might be rated as satisfactory in a seventy-five year old. It is not uncommon for various aspects of a person's physical health to be compared with averages for persons in his or her own age group.

The older individual also makes judgments about whether his or her health is satisfactory. Some older individuals rate their health as quite satisfactory, even though a physician could point to actions that could be taken to improve it. When asked about the state of their health, it is not uncommon for older persons to reply, "Pretty good for someone my age." By making this statement, they are suggesting that their standard for good health is somewhat less demanding than it would be if they were younger. Unfortunately, sometimes older persons attribute problems that can be remedied to "normal" aging. Health workers who serve older persons are particularly interested in providing health education to help older persons learn that many of the problems that they accept as part of the aging process are amenable to treatment. Even when older persons are aware of measures that could improve their health, they may be reluctant to take these measures. They are, in effect, rating their current state of health as satisfactory when compared with the cost (in time, money, effort, or pain) of improving it. One example of this is obesity, which is believed to increase the risk of hypertension and heart disease and to contribute to the severity of arthritis. People may be well aware of the potential health benefits of controlled weight loss but choose not to lose weight because they perceive their current health as satisfactory when compared with the difficulties of reducing. On the opposite side, some older persons rate their health as unsatisfactory when their physicians can find no physiological basis for their complaints.

Satisfactory health is a relative concept. It lies, in part, in the eye of the beholder. One's assessment of a person's health status is affected by whether one is comparing a person's current health to an ideal standard, to his or her health in previous years, to the health of other people the same age, or to the state of health that the person would like to attain and is willing to work toward. As helping professionals, we would like to work toward the goal of helping all older persons attain a state of health that is satisfactory to them. Some older persons are unaware of ways in which their health can be improved. Others will choose not to take measures likely to improve their health. Still others will not be able to afford to improve their health status because of limited financial resources.

What Is the Health Status of Older Americans?

Generally, older Americans assess their health as quite good. A 1982 survey conducted by the National Center for Health Statistics found that 65 percent of noninstitutionalized older persons rated their own health as excellent, very good, or good, when compared with others their own age (U.S. Senate Special Committee on Aging, 1984). In another study, when simply asked whether they rated their health as excellent, good, only fair, or poor, 17 percent rated their health as excellent and another 39 percent rated it as good (Lou Harris and Associates, 1981). In this same study only 21 percent of elderly respondents saw poor health as a serious personal problem, although 47 percent of persons aged eighteen to sixty-four believed that poor health was a very serious problem for most people over sixty-five. Clearly, the young believe older people suffer health problems to a far greater extent than older people themselves believe is the case.

At the same time, it is well known that physiological aging (senescence) brings with it increased vulnerability to disease and death. Older persons use physicians more often than younger persons, enter hospitals more frequently and stay longer, and use more prescription drugs. They are far more likely to need institutional care, although at any given time only about 5 percent of the older population is institutionalized.

Generally, older persons suffer from chronic health problems more frequently than from acute illnesses. Approximately 80 percent of those sixty-five and older have at least one chronic illness, but only about 20 percent must limit their activities because of their condition. The top five chronic problems experienced by the elderly are arthritis, hypertension, hearing impairments, heart conditions, and orthopedic impairments, in that order. We shall discuss the implications of these impairments later in this chapter.

Tremendous advances in health care technology have been made during the lifetime of our current older population. Average life expectancy at birth in 1900 was forty-seven years; in 1983 it was seventy-five years (U.S. Senate Special Committee on Aging, 1985). These gains in life expectancy, however, primarily reflect our successes in preventing and curing acute illnesses, thus reducing deaths that formerly occurred in childhood and young adulthood. A result is that people who might have died at younger ages in the past are now living to advanced age and are at risk for the chronic problems and diseases that do not usually manifest themselves until after age fifty. The challenge of promoting successful aging now and in the future will be caring for a large population of older persons with chronic health problems.

Common Health Problems

In this section we discuss briefly many of the health problems that are common in old age. Much of the information presented here is based on a continuing series of publications of the National Institute on Aging called *Age Pages*. Designed primarily for the older consumer of health care services, they are invaluable references for older persons and those who work with them. Although we cannot hope to provide more than a cursory overview of older persons' health concerns in one short chapter, we believe that it is most important for human service professionals to have a good working knowledge of the problems older persons confront. Readers are urged to consult more comprehensive works for more detailed information.

Problems with Vision

Generally speaking, older people have more trouble with their eyes than younger persons, but most maintain good eyesight until quite late in life. Most people experience a gradual decline in the ability to focus on small print or to see close objects clearly as they grow older. This condition, known as presbyopia, is what leads people to hold the telephone book at arm's length in order to read it. The condition can be corrected with glasses. Older persons may also suffer from loss of color vision. Because the lens of the eye tends to yellow with advancing age, it filters out the violets, blues, and greens of the color spectrum. Thus, older persons generally have a much easier time seeing yellow, red, and orange than the darker colors. This should be borne in mind by professionals involved in designing environments where older persons spend a great deal of time. An environment designed with bright colors is much more likely to provide visual stimulation than one decorated in the darker peaceful tones. Also, since the older eye admits less light, it is helpful to provide sufficient illumination in spaces where older persons will be reading or doing close work.

A common eye disease in old age is cataracts. Cataracts are the result of a gradual opaque or filmy buildup in the lens. When a person has cataracts, light is diffused, and the person is particularly sensitive to glare. Substantial visual impairment may occur. Fortunately, cataracts can be removed surgically, and cataract operations are almost always successful. Older persons who have had cataract surgery are frequently amazed at the extent of their improved vision.

Older persons may also suffer from glaucoma. This condition results from a buildup of fluid and pressure in the eye and can result in blindness. Because a person may be unaware of this condition until damage is done, it is important to have regular eye checkups, including tests for glaucoma. Treatment may include medication, special eyedrops, or surgery.

The National Institute on Aging recommends that older persons have regular health checkups so that physical conditions that may affect the eyes (diabetes, high blood pressure) can be detected early and treated. They also suggest eye examinations every two or three years to check on prescriptions for glasses and to test for the presence of eye disease.

Professionals should be aware that visual impairments may influence older persons' activities and opportunities. Because many older persons' eyes do not adapt well to dark, the elderly are often reluctant to drive at night. Activities scheduled after dark to which older persons must drive are not likely to be well attended. Many older persons prefer to read the large print books that are available at most public libraries. Service personnel should take care that forms and brochures that they design for older persons are printed in sufficiently large type to be seen by someone with impaired vision. Environments for older persons should be designed bearing in mind the way color vision changes with age. Finally, professionals must remember that hesitancy in older persons with whom they work may be the result of difficulties in seeing, not slowness of mind or lack of motivation.

Problems with Hearing

Hearing loss is a common problem in old age. Some 30 percent of persons sixty-five to seventy-four and fifty percent of those seventy-five to seventy-nine have some degree of hearing loss. Loss of hearing is a particularly vexing problem, because it results in limitations in communication and social interactions. When older persons cannot hear what others are saying, they may become suspicious of them. Paranoid symptoms may develop as a result of hearing impairment. Older (and younger) persons with hearing loss are often perceived by others to be stupid, confused, or unresponsive. Friends and relatives become frustrated with older persons who are afraid to admit they cannot hear well and do not seek help that may alleviate the problem.

One type of hearing impairment, presbycusis, results in the inability to hear speech clearly enough. Changes in the inner ear make it difficult for the person to hear certain types of sounds. Typically, this type of hearing loss begins with the inability to hear higher frequencies (consonant sounds), while the ability to hear lower frequencies (vowel sounds) remains unaffected. Under these conditions, speech sounds are garbled, and it is difficult for the hearer to make sense of what is being said. Shouting at a person suffering from presbycusis does not help the problem, because all that is heard is loud, unintelligible sounds—a most unpleasant experience for the hearer! The best way to talk with someone with presbycusis is to lower the pitch of one's voice while still speaking clearly and at sufficient volume.

A second type of hearing impairment is the inability to hear speech loudly enough. This may be the result of conduction deafness, a condition in which blockage or impairment keeps sound waves from traveling through the ear normally. Conduction deafness can be treated by flushing the ear (to clear out packed ear wax), medication, or surgery. Inability to hear speech loudly enough may also be the result of central deafness (damage to the nerve centers in the brain). Central deafness may be caused by illness, drugs, exposure to loud noise over a long period of time, head injury, or other causes. This condition, which affects how language is understood, cannot be cured. Work with an audiologist or speech therapist may help the sufferer cope more satisfactorily.

Those working with older persons who appear to suffer from an untreated hearing loss should urge them to seek diagnosis and treatment. Health and social service personnel must bear in mind that paranoia, confusion, depression, and unresponsiveness among the elderly often have their root in hearing impairments. Often, hearing impairments can be alleviated with proper treatment. In addition, older persons with hearing losses can be encouraged to request that others repeat what they didn't hear clearly and to modify background noise in situations where they want to be sure they hear what is being said.

Professionals should bear in mind that many of the older persons they work with will have some degree of hearing impairment. They should get in the habit of speaking clearly, without shouting or over-articulating their words. Since visual cues take on added importance to the hearing impaired person, it is important to position oneself near enough so one can be seen clearly. One should avoid chewing, covering one's mouth, or turning away when speaking to a hearing impaired person. Whenever possible, choose a place for conversation that is quiet and where little background noise will intrude.

Skeletomuscular Problems

The most common, chronic health problem of older persons is arthritis. This condition can be very painful and seriously affect the ability of older persons to move about freely and go about the business of daily living. Arthritis involves problems with joints. Two types of arthritis are common among older persons. The first, osteoarthritis, is a degenerative disease, apparently related to wear and tear on the body's joints. Heredity and obesity may also contribute to one's likelihood of suffering from osteoarthritis. Almost all older persons suffer from osteoarthritis to some degree, and it is most likely to affect the knees, hips, and spine. Those with this condition experience pain and stiffness, occasionally resulting in considerable disability.

The more serious and disabling type of arthritis is rheumatoid arthritis. This condition, which is much more common in women than in men, is the result of the inflammation of a joint membrane. The joints become swollen and painful. If untreated, severe damage to the joints may occur, resulting in crippling. Rheumatoid arthritis is not limited to old age, but many people age with the disease.

The most commonly prescribed treatment for arthritis is aspirin. This is known to reduce inflammation and to reduce pain. Because large doses of aspirin are often used, it is important that persons with arthritis take aspirin under medical supervision, because aspirin may have undesirable side effects. With professional advice, arthritis sufferers can develop an appropriate physical regimen that usually involves a balance between exercise and rest.

Arthritis is an often painful and frustrating condition that affects millions of older persons. Unfortunately, arthritis sufferers have become the targets of unscrupulous persons marketing "cures." Hundreds of millions of dollars a year are spent on products that have dubious benefits. The National Institute on Aging warns older persons against drugs, diets, or mechanical devices that promise quick or miracle cures or relief from arthritis. Using drugs prescribed or recommended by a physician, together with physical therapy, is the best course of action for those seeking relief from arthritis.

Another condition affecting the skeletal system of older persons is osteoporosis. Osteoporosis, a condition in which bone mass becomes thinner over a long number of years, affects one quarter of women over the age of sixty. It is believed that loss of bone tissue may result from decreasing hormone levels, not getting enough calcium, inadequate exposure to sunlight, and inactivity. The gradual loss of bone mass may be asymptomatic and thus go undetected for years. In later life, however, sufferers may experience frequent fractures, backache, and slumped posture. In extreme cases, the person suffering from osteoporosis will have a severe curving of the spine (dowager's hump) and will break bones by merely stretching or bending. Once the condition is diagnosed, physicians concentrate on preventing further bone loss.

Considerable attention is being paid to the prevention of osteoporosis. Fair-skinned, white women with small frames are most at risk. Physicians currently recommend that younger women be sure to get enough calcium and vitamin D and that they engage in regular exercise as a preventive measure.

Older persons frequently suffer from persistent lower back pain, a chronic problem that may be related to injury, disease, or poor posture. Temporary episodes of acute pain may be brought on by sudden twisting or turning or incorrect lifting. These episodes can last days to months. Good posture habits, coupled with sensible approaches to lifting, can help prevent or alleviate back problems. One should sit in chairs that provide appropriate support for the curve in the lower back and one should rest on a firm mattress. A firm pillow placed in the small of the back is recommended for those expecting to sit for a long time in the same position (for example, automobile trips). Stretching exercises are frequently recommended. Muscle relaxants and rest are often prescribed for those experiencing acutely painful episodes.

Generally, older persons have less muscle mass and muscle strength than younger persons. Muscle-wasting diseases, however, occur more commonly in young and middle-aged adults. It is believed that at least some loss of muscle mass and functioning among the old is the result of lack of use. Regular exercise, at a level appropriate for the older person's physical condition, is recommended to retain or regain feelings of health and vigor.

Conditions Affecting the Heart and Circulatory System

The second most common chronic condition among older adults is hypertension, often called high blood pressure. In persons with high blood pressure, the blood exerts a higher than normal amount of pressure against the blood vessels as it is pumped out of the heart. Although this may produce no symptoms noticeable to the person who has it, the result can be catastrophic. Hypertension is often called the silent killer and those who have it are at risk for stroke, heart failure, and kidney disease. The causes of hypertension are unknown, but it is associated with arteriosclerotic and atherosclerotic conditions, obesity, high salt intake, and lack of exercise. Hypertension appears to run in families, and blacks are more likely to suffer from it than whites.

The term *hypertension* leads some people mistakenly to believe that the condition is caused by tenseness or nervousness. This is not the case. Although in all of us blood pressure becomes elevated when we are under stress or engage in strenuous activity, one can suffer from hypertension even if one is usually a calm, relaxed person.

Fortunately, hypertension can be controlled by medication. Most people diagnosed with hypertension need to take medication for the rest of their lives. It is important that they continue to take the medication as prescribed even if they are feeling good. Some hypertension medications have undesirable side effects, including impotence and frequent urination. These should be reported to one's physician, since a different medication without the undesired side effect can often be substituted. Many health facilities provide free or low-cost screening clinics for hypertension for older persons. A blood pressure check is painless and takes little time. Regular blood pressure checks should be part of every older person's health routine.

One of the leading causes of death among older persons is heart and vascular disease. One such condition is atherosclerosis, the buildup of fatty substances on the inside walls of the blood vessels. When one has this condition, blood flow is obstructed, and the heart must work harder. In some cases, blood flow to an area of the body may be totally closed off. If blood flow to the heart is restricted, a heart attack may occur. Insufficient blood going to the brain can result in a stroke. Atherosclerosis is thought to result from a diet that contains too much animal fat. It has also been associated with cigarette smoking, lack of exercise, obesity, and heredity. Persons suffering from atherosclerosis can sometimes be treated surgically, with diseased blood vessels replaced or bypassed.

Arteriosclerosis refers to the hardening or loss of elasticity of the blood vessels. This, too, results in loss of blood flow. Blood-thinning medication may be prescribed for persons with both atherosclerosis and arteriosclerosis.

Both atherosclerosis and arteriosclerosis contribute to heart disease. Many older persons suffer from angina pains, a feeling of pressure in the chest, loss of breath, and burning sensations, resulting from reduced blood flow. Reduced blood flow to the heart may result in myocardial infarct (heart attack), a condition in which part of the heart tissue dies from lack of blood. Symptoms of a heart attack include pain in the chest, shoulder, or left arm, although some heart attacks are silent and unnoticed. The person suffering a heart attack may experience nausea, fainting, and general weakness. If sufficient damage occurs, the heart attack victim will die. Medication, a change in diet, cessation of smoking, and an exercise regime are frequently prescribed for survivors. In some cases, surgery is used to bypass clogged arteries.

Congestive heart failure is the impaired pumping efficiency of the heart. Many conditions may strain the heart, resulting in congestive heart failure. Among them are atherosclerosis, arteriosclerosis, hypertension, impaired blood flow to the kidneys, and previous heart attacks. Medication, changes in activity patterns, weight reduction, and reduction in sodium in the diet are typically advised.

Cardiovascular diseases are often serious and severely disabling. At the same time, with proper supervision and the involvement of the patient in his or her treatment, they can be managed successfully for many years. Many persons with cardiovascular diseases live satisfactory and relatively normal lives. The professional who works with such persons may find it necessary to help them cope with the depression that may accompany limitations.

Cerebrovascular Problems

When there is a sudden disruption of the flow of blood to an area of the brain a cerebrovascular accident (or stroke) is said to have occurred. The result is that the cells in the brain, deprived of blood during the CVA, are damaged or die, and the bodily processes controlled by those cells may be damaged, temporarily or permanently. Strokes may occur for several different reasons. A thrombotic stroke can occur when atherosclerotic deposits build up on an artery that supplies blood to the brain. Initially, blood flow is just slowed. Eventually a clot or lump may block passage of the blood entirely. An embolic stroke occurs when fatty deposits built up elsewhere in the body break off, travel to the brain, and lodge in the cerebral arteries. Here again, circulation to some area of the brain is closed off. Finally, hemorrhagic strokes are caused when a cerebral blood vessel bursts, spurting blood into areas of the brain where it was not intended to go.

The effects of stroke can vary widely, depending upon how much of and what part of the brain is affected. A severe stroke can result in death. In other cases, the patient survives but will be left with some impairment. Paralysis on one side of the body is common, with the side opposite the site of the stroke being affected. When there is injury to the left side of the brain, the right side of the body is most affected. Speech and language are likely to be impaired, and the patient's behavioral style following the stroke may be slow and cautious. Persons suffering damage to the right side of the brain are likely to have paralysis on the left side of the body. They will often have difficulty with spatial-perceptual tasks such as judging distance, size, and rate of movement. They may tend to be impulsive or careless and believe their capacities are greater than they are.

Rehabilitation following stroke usually begins while the patient is still hospitalized. Physical therapy is generally important in helping the patient strengthen muscles and learn to move with mechanical aids. Speech and language therapy are prescribed for those whose ability to communicate orally has been impaired. Drugs are prescribed to prevent the occurrence of further strokes. Rehabilitation from a stroke can be a slow, challenging process. It is important to give positive reinforcement for the hard work patients do in learning to walk or speak again after brain injury. Family members need special guidance in understanding changed behavior patterns and in providing support that will contribute to recovery.

The conditions that lead to stroke develop over many years. Considerable efforts are now being made to prevent stroke before it occurs. Generally, the same measures taken to prevent cardiovascular disease will also reduce the likelihood of stroke. These include control of high blood pressure, cessation of cigarette smoking, eating a diet low in animal fat, getting regular exercise, and controlling diabetes. Persons who have suffered brief, strokelike symptoms (for example, temporary numbness, difficulty with speech, momentary blindness, unexplained headaches) are at particular risk for stroke. These brief symptoms may be transient ischemic attacks (TIA's) and should be reported immediately to one's physician. Medication to regulate blood pressure or to thin the blood, coupled with lifestyle changes, can avert a stroke in persons who are at risk.

Gastrointestinal Problems

The gastrointestinal system consists of those parts of the body involved in the intake, processing and digestion, and elimination of food. Problems that occur in one part of the system can affect functioning of other parts of the system. In this section, we deal briefly with conditions in various parts of the gastrointestinal tract that are often troublesome for older persons.

Proper digestion begins with effective chewing and lubrication of the food in the mouth. Unfortunately, many older persons suffer from poor oral health that impedes these processes. Due to poor nutritional and dental practices in the past, lack of funds for dental care, and the erroneous belief that it is "normal" to lose teeth with advancing age, over 40 percent of older Americans have lost all of their own teeth by age sixty-five. Many have ill-fitting dentures that cause sores, inefficient chewing, and embarrassment. It is important for older persons to be aware of good oral hygiene practices, including the brushing and cleaning of dentures. Also, regular dental checkups are important in old age, even if the older person has dentures. Dentists can check for gum disease, oral cancer, and sores in the mouth. They can advise on how to cope with a frequent complaint among older persons, persistent feelings of dryness in the mouth. In addition to working with diseased teeth, they can repair or replace dentures. Unfortunately, many people place a low priority on dental care. Few health insurance programs available to the old (or the young) pay for dental care. One result has been that problems that could have been prevented or treated in earlier years persist and become more severe in later life.

Some older persons suffer from difficulty with swallowing, heartburn, and other conditions associated with the esophagus (tube running from the mouth to the stomach). Hiatal hernia (a condition where a section of the upper part of the stomach bulges through the diaphragm) can lead to pain and a feeling of fullness. It is quite common in old age, particularly among women who are overweight. Weight reduction, eating smaller, more frequent meals, and resting with the upper body elevated may bring relief. Persons with this condition are urged to avoid coffee, tea, alcohol, and before-bedtime snacks. A burning sensation in the upper chest described as heartburn results from stomach acids entering and remaining in the esophagus. Medication may be recommended, as well as weight reduction and avoiding eating for several hours before bed.

Older persons may suffer from a variety of problems with the stomach or small intestine, resulting in pain, vomiting, constipation, gas, and distension of the abdomen. Persons with these symptoms should consult a physician promptly. Many are fearful that their symptoms are indicative of cancer, when, in fact, ulcers, intestinal obstructions, gastritis, or diet may be the cause.

Gallbladder problems are not uncommon among older persons. The gallbladder is a small organ located below the liver. Its function is to store and secrete bile, a substance used in the digestive process. Some older persons develop gallstones that build up from salts in the bile. These can result in pain, nausea, and vomiting. In some cases, physicians choose to remove the gallstones surgically; in others they concentrate on medical management, which may include use of antacids and avoidance of fatty foods.

Many older persons fear they have constipation and other conditions associated with the large intestine. The primary function of the large intestine is to store food wastes and move them toward elimination. Many older persons become concerned about whether their large intestine is functioning properly. Complaints about constipation may occur with changes in the frequency of bowel movements, painful or difficult passage of stools, or the passage of blood.

A number of serious problems with the functioning of the large intestine are possible, and older persons are urged to consult candidly with their physicians about problems they are experiencing. Despite what many of today's older persons were taught in their youth, it is not necessary to have a daily bowel movement to be in good health. The regular use of over-the-counter laxatives or enemas is strongly discouraged since it can become habit forming and may result in poor absorption of vitamins or an upset in the body's electrolyte balance. The symptoms of constipation may be treated successfully by adding more bulk and fiber to the diet, drinking more liquids, and getting more exercise.

Problems with bowel functioning may be caused by colo-rectal cancer, the most common cancer among those over seventy. Although survival rates following early detection are high, far fewer Americans are aware of this disease than they are of other forms of cancer. Regular checks for colo-rectal cancer could add years to the lives of older Americans.

Diverticular disease is quite common among older persons. This results from inflammation in areas of the bowel wall. Persons with this problem may suffer from pain, diarrhea, constipation, and bleeding.

Usually a high-fiber diet is prescribed along with the use of antibiotic drugs.

Hemorrhoids (ruptured blood vessels in the area of the anus) are common among older persons. In some cases they present no problems; in others, they may bleed and/or be very painful. Severe hemorrhoids are often removed surgically. In other cases, a diet with increased bulk and drinking more water is prescribed. Persons with rectal problems are urged to seek medical advice before treating suspected hemorrhoids with over-the-counter medications, since the symptoms they are experiencing may be associated with a more serious condition.

Respiratory Problems

Older persons may suffer from both acute and chronic problems with the respiratory system. Like people of all ages, they may suffer from the common cold or from various influenza viruses. Unlike younger people, however, their symptoms may be more severe and last longer. These acute illnesses may also lower the older person's resistance, leaving him or her prey to more serious infections including pneumonia. For these reasons, older persons are urged to take special precautions to avoid acute respiratory infections. Influenza, a viral infection of the nose, throat, and lungs that can result in weakness, cough, headache, chills, fever and muscle aches can be prevented by vaccination. Persons sixty-five and older are encouraged to get an annual flu vaccination. Physicians may prescribe an antiviral drug for persons particularly at risk.

Pneumonia, a bacterial inflammation of the lungs, is a leading cause of death among older persons. Symptoms are similar to those of flu, but more severe. Treatment usually consists of antibiotic drugs and introduction of extra liquids.

Chronic bronchitis and emphysema are known collectively as chronic obstructive lung disease. This condition develops slowly and can cause serious limitations in middle and old age. Unfortunately, by the time the condition presents noticeable symptoms, severe damage may have already been done. Damage to the bronchial tubes and lungs from infection or exposure to dust or cigarette smoke leads to a condition characterized by chronic coughing, chronic expectoration, and shortness of breath. The airway may become irritated and obstructed. Persons with chronic obstructive lung disease have sustained permanent, irreparable damage to respiratory tissue. After diagnosis, efforts are made to prevent or slow further damage through the reduction or cessation of cigarette smoking. Sufferers are encouraged to take part in rehabilitation programs that help them more efficiently use the lung capacity they have remaining. Oxygen may be prescribed. Since respiratory infections are particularly dangerous for chronic obstructive lung disease patients, special care is taken to avoid exposure to cold or flu viruses.

Lung cancer is a major cause of death in older persons. Unfortunately, by the time lung cancer is diagnosed, there is very little that can be done to slow the progress of the disease. Most lung cancers are caused by cigarette smoking. Primarily a disease found in men in the past, lung cancer is now being diagnosed in increasing numbers of women.

Many older smokers are aware of the dangers of this habit. They know that they are at greater risk of developing incurable pulmonary problems, heart disease, and stroke, but believe that they are too old for quitting smoking to do any good. The National Institute on Aging points out that, while it is true that stopping smoking will not reverse permanent damage already done, risks for heart disease and lung cancer decline among those who do stop. Since smokers have greater chances of getting respiratory illnesses, stopping smoking can reduce the number of days a person is sick with these ailments. Older smokers may also be motivated to quit by recent evidence of the damage second-hand smoke may do to the nonsmokers in their environment. Regardless of one's age or how long one has smoked, there are health benefits to stopping smoking.

Skin Problems

Probably the most easily identifiable physical changes that occur in later life are those in the skin. As people age, their skin tends to become wrinkled and dry. Some degree of elasticity is lost with the loss of fat directly beneath the skin. One result of this loss of fat is that older persons become more sensitive to both heat and cold. Many older persons experience change in the skin pigmentation, with some areas of the skin losing color and dark spots appearing on other parts. The loss of pigmentary cells in the hair results in the graying characteristic of old age.

Older persons may suffer from a number of skin disorders including eczema and psoriasis. Those who have spent a great deal of time out of doors are susceptible to skin cancers, lesions that physicians typically burn off or remove surgically.

For some, the problems caused by changes in the skin are more important psychologically than medically. Wrinkles, graying hair, "age spots," and a sagging chin are dreaded because they may suggest a lack of vigor. Persons reluctant to identify themselves as aging or old may go to great lengths to disguise changes in their skin or hair. Others, perhaps more accepting of aging, point to their wrinkles and gray hair with pride, noting that they earned them!

It is not uncommon for older persons to report problems with their feet. While foot problems are generally not life-threatening, they can cause considerable discomfort and limit mobility. As is the case with younger people, the old may suffer from a number of fungal and bacterial infections causing peeling, itching, and blisters. These can lead to infections that are difficult to cure. Warts are growths on the skin caused by viruses and can be removed surgically or burned or "frozen" off. Corns and callouses generally result from friction and rubbing against shoes, but may be caused by a bone deformity. Bunions occur when joints in the toes become unaligned, swell, and become tender. When a toenail grows through the skin of the toe, one is said to have an ingrown toenail. This may occur because the nails have been improperly trimmed. The result may be an infection at the point where the nail pierces the skin.

Persons with other health problems may find that these problems affect their feet. For example, persons with atherosclerosis or diabetes may develop sores on their feet that are extremely difficult to heal. Because injuries to the feet can be particularly dangerous for diabetics, those suffering from this disease should get immediate medical attention if their feet are cut. Older persons who have trouble trimming their toenails (diabetics in particular) should get professional assistance to prevent injury.

Older persons experiencing problems with their feet should consult their physician or a podiatrist (health professional who diagnoses, treats, and prevents diseases of the foot). Often medication or surgery can alleviate the distress. Generally, older persons should take actions that improve circulation to the feet. This includes exercise, massage, and warm foot baths. It is particularly important in old age to choose shoes that are safe, comfortable, and give the feet opportunity to breathe.

Reproductive System Problems

Although women past the menopause cannot bear children, older women and men can and do enjoy sexuality unless an illness or injury interferes. Men in their eighties have been known to father children.

Women experience menopausal changes in their fourth or fifth decade. As a result of normal hormonal changes, menstrual cycles become irregular and eventually cease, and the female no longer is capable of conception. During a period that may last as long as two to three years, the body gradually changes, sometimes producing symptoms of overheating known as hot flashes. For most women, these changes do not result in major problems, either physiological or psychological.

Postmenopausal women are likely to experience a thinning and drying of the vaginal wall that can make sexual intercourse painful. Also, loss of subcutaneous fat in the area of the external genitalia and loss of hormones can lead to pain or inflammation. Despite these changes, women can be fully sexually responsive well into the seventies. Women experiencing pain with sexual activity should consult their physicians, since the use of medications and lubricants has been found to alleviate these problems.

In men, the level of sperm production decreases with advancing age, as does the the production of male hormones. Barring injury or disease, aged men remain capable of sexual intercourse to climax well into their later years. They are, however, likely to notice some changes from their younger years. It will likely take them longer to achieve an erection, but they will be able to maintain it longer. The orgasmic phase of intercourse is likely to be briefer, and they will experience a longer refractory time (time until they can get an erection again).

Many people fear a loss in their sexual capabilities with advancing age. Men, for example, may experience an episode of impotence and mistakenly believe their sexual life is over forever. Usually, impotence in older men is caused by the same factors that promote it in younger men: fear of failure, overindulgence in food or alcohol, depression, tension, and anxiety. Men with concern about their potency should consult frankly with their physicians. Although there may be an underlying physiological cause (for example, diabetes, side effects of medication), men can usually be reassured that they can remain sexually active well into late life.

Human service professionals need to be aware that a person's interest in love, affection, and sexual intimacy does not diminish merely because he or she has grown old. Interest in another as a love and sexual partner is as natural and normal among older adults as it is among younger adults. When an older adult shows a romantic interest in another person, it should be treated as neither scandalous nor cute but as a normal adult response to the need for intimacy.

Urinary System Problems

Older persons may experience a number of problems with their urinary systems. Urinary tract infections may occur, resulting in burning sensations, increased need to urinate at night, and the sense of having to urinate frequently. If acute, these infections can generally be cleared up with drug therapy. Chronic urinary tract infections may be related to an obstruction in the system and are considerably more difficult to treat. Older persons may also suffer from inflammation of the kidneys (pyelonephritis) and from the development of kidney stones.

Men may experience problems having their origin with the prostate gland, an organ about the size of a walnut that surrounds the urethra (tube that carries urine from the body). In some men the prostate gland becomes infected, resulting in chills, fever, painful urination, and lower back pain. Some may suffer from an enlarged prostate gland that obstructs the flow of urine through the urethra. This can cause difficulty with urination and incomplete voiding. In severe cases, surgery may be performed to remove areas of the prostate that are causing the obstruction. Surgery to correct an enlarged prostate has no physiological effect on a man's ability to engage in sexual activity.

Urinary incontinence is a difficult and embarrassing problem that affects over 10 percent of older Americans, at least to some degree. Generally, incontinence refers to passing urine in an undesired situation, and may describe the leakage of urine that may occur during laughing, sneezing, or coughing, the leakage from a constantly filled bladder (for example, in a man whose urethra is blocked by an enlarged prostate gland) or the severe wetting that may occur when one is unable to hold urine long enough to reach a toilet. Incontinence can be caused by a number of factors, among them stretching of tissue during childbirth, blockage or other disorder of the urinary system, or the effects of other conditions (including stroke, Alzheimer's disease, stupor produced by strong drugs). Treatment varies depending on the factors that are causing the problem. Medication and exercises may be prescribed, and in some cases surgery can be helpful. Some behavioral management techniques have been helpful, as has been the implantation of prosthetic devices. Unfortunately, regaining continence is unrealistic for some persons and the use of catheters, collecting devices, or absorbent underclothing is recommended.

Diabetes

Diabetes mellitus is a condition in which the body's ability to control the level of glucose (the digestive by-product of sugars and starches) in the blood is impaired. When the amount of glucose in the body is too high or too low, damage may occur to numerous body organs. Some people have diabetes from childhood on. Others develop it in middle or old age. Predisposing factors for diabetes are a history of diabetes in the family or being overweight. Symptoms of diabetes may be vague, and include feelings of fatigue, unusual thirst, frequent urination, blurring of vision, skin infections, difficulty with healing, and unusual weight loss. Physicians diagnose diabetes using tests for sugar in the urine or blood.

There is no cure for diabetes but it can be controlled. Those with more severe diabetes can control it with the use of insulin, careful attention to diet, and an exercise program. Some diabetes sufferers, however, do not need to use insulin to control their blood glucose. Weight reduction, careful diet, and daily exercise are typical approaches to treatment. Since diabetics are susceptible to numerous other conditions, it is vital that they learn to pay careful attention to their bodies. Adherence to the prescribed treatment regime, together with meticulous care of the feet and skin, is important. Also, the diabetic should report promptly changes in vision and mobility that may occur. Patients should be made aware of the warning signs of very high and low blood sugar so that they can take adequate precautions and get immediate medical attention if necessary.

Although diabetes is a chronic illness that requires considerable patient participation in its successful management, it need not interfere with normal living.

Sleep Problems

Older people frequently report, as do younger people, difficulties with getting a good night's rest. The National Institute on Aging reports that sleep disturbance is a frequent problem of older adults. There are many causes of sleep disturbance. One, prevalent among the old, is sleep apnea, a temporary halt in breathing that may last from a few seconds to a minute or more. Typically, the person awakens during an incident of apnea, resumes normal breathing, and is unaware that there ever was a problem. Older individuals may experience scores to hundreds of apneas in a single night, resulting in less than restful sleep. Sleep apnea can be dangerous, particularly if older persons also take sleeping pills. Since these depress breathing, the possibility arises of not awakening when breathing stops. Sleep researchers have found that periods of sleep apnea are associated with brief, sharp rises in blood pressure, even for persons with normal daytime blood pressure. These episodes may, in turn, be associated with heart disease and stroke.

Sleep disturbances may also be caused by other conditions. Many older persons suffer from leg twitches during the night that can awaken them. The use of caffeine, pain, the need to get up to urinate at night, use of drugs and alcohol, and depression or emotional disturbance can affect sleep.

Although sleeping pills are prescribed for many older individuals (particularly those in institutions), the National Institute on Aging recommends against their long-term use. Since older persons tend to use many drugs anyway, the chance exists that sleeping pills will interact negatively with other medications. Older persons process drugs more slowly than the young, and the active agents in sleeping pills may build up over a period of time, having negative effects on movement, alertness, and functioning during the day. Long-term use may increase rather than decrease sleep disturbance.

Generally, a natural approach to getting a good night's rest is recommended. This includes going to bed when one is tired, sleeping in a dark, quiet room, and avoiding alcohol, caffeine, heavy meals, cigarettes, and strenuous exercise before going to bed. To relax, a warm glass of milk or a soothing bath is suggested. Persons with persistent sleep problems should consult their physicians.

Alcohol and Drugs

Misuse and overuse of alcohol and drugs cause problems for older as well as younger persons. Alcohol abusers in late life fall into two categories: persons who have been heavy drinkers for a long time and those who begin drinking heavily in late life in response to life changes. Chronic alcoholics often die before they reach old age, and those who reach later life are likely to have suffered damage to their brain, central nervous system, liver, heart, stomach, and kidneys. Those who begin alcohol and drug abuse in later life are often reacting to negative life circumstances: death of spouse or friends, decline in income, boredom following retirement, or poor health.

Although the moderate use of alcohol may have beneficial effects throughout adult life, excessive use can be devastating. In addition to its assault on various parts of the body, alcohol abuse impairs coordination and judgment, making the abuser prone to accidents. Excessive use of alcohol can mask other physiological symptoms, delaying the diagnosis and treatment of heart disease and other illnesses. Alcohol intoxication can lead to symptoms of dementia, resulting in unneeded nursing home placement. Finally, alcohol interacts with a number of medications that may be prescribed for older persons, influencing their effect. Even those who drink moderately should be candid with their physicians about the amount they drink to avoid potential drug interaction effects.

It is difficult to arrest a drinking problem without the active co-operation of the drinker. Some people find that inpatient programs that provide medical detoxification as well as behavioral and psychosocial therapy are necessary. Others find that they can stop drinking with the help of outpatient organizations (for example, Alcoholics Anonymous). Older problem drinkers generally do well in treatment programs once they have made the decision that they want to stop abusing.

Older adults rarely use illegal drugs. They may, however, suffer from drug abuse problems by attempting to medicate themselves without supervision. Drug abuse problems may occur when an older person uses medications prescribed for someone else, makes heavy, regular use of over-the-counter medications (e.g., laxatives) without consulting health personnel, or alters dosages of prescribed medications. The interaction of certain drugs with one another or the interaction of drugs with certain foods can produce life-threatening effects, making self-medication potentially dangerous. Older persons should always tell their physicians about all drugs (prescribed and over the counter) that they are taking to avoid negative interaction effects.

Cancer

Older persons are often concerned, with good reason, about being diagnosed with cancer. Cancer is one of the three leading causes of death among the elderly. There are many different types of cancer, each with different symptoms and potential for recovery. Generally, cancer is a disease in which cells grow abnormally, invading healthy tissue and starving the normal parts of the body of nutrition. If unchecked, cancer will spread, leading to death.

The most common sites of cancer among the old are in the lung, breast, colon and rectum, prostate (for men), reproductive organs (for women), and on the skin. It is recommended that persons have regular screening checks for developing cancers beginning at about age fifty. These include rectal exams and analysis of stool samples, pelvic exams, pap smears, breast exams and mammographs for women, and prompt attention to changes in warts or moles. Anyone who coughs persistently, experiences shortness of breath, or spits up blood should be checked immediately for lung cancer.

It was once the case that a cancer diagnosis meant death within a short period of time. Now, chances for survival are better than they have ever been for those whose cancer is detected early. Depending on the site and extent of the cancer, treatment may include chemotherapy, radiation, and/or surgery to remove the cancerous cells and prevent their spread. Many older persons can be successfully treated for cancer and live normally and productively for many years. For others, the prognosis is not so good. Treatment can be painful, disfiguring, and exhausting with little hope offered for significant extension of life. In some of these cases, patients choose treatment whose goal is alleviation of pain rather than extension of life.

Resources for Health Care

Throughout this chapter we have stressed the importance of good health practices to prevent problems common in old age or to catch them in the early stages when they are most amenable to treatment. Some problems that occur late in life have their origins in youth and early adulthood, suggesting that prevention should begin early. Older persons of the future will be spared many of the health problems today's elderly suffer from if they adopt a way of living that includes early and regular care of the teeth and gums, regular physical activity, a nutritious diet low in animal fat, avoidance of cigarette smoking, and regular visits to physicians and other health professionals to check for early symptoms of problems.

It is astounding to think of the advances in medical knowledge and treatment that have occurred during the lifetime of today's seventy-five year olds. We now know much more specifically about the dangers of smoking, poor diet, and inactivity. We are able to cure easily conditions that were essentially untreatable in the past, and we can prevent diseases from taking hold through the use of vaccine. Unfortunately, many of today's older persons were unable to take advantage of this knowledge in time to prevent the problems from which they now suffer. Even now, some remain unaware or unable to make use of the resources available to improve the quality of their current health. To many, today's health care facilities are bewildering and threatening. Lack of knowledge about what is available, fear of the cost of health care, and fear of learning one has a dread disease serve as barriers to many older persons' regular use of health care professionals. Efforts at health education for the elderly should focus not only on good personal health practices, but also on appropriate use of health care resources in their community.

Preventive Care

One way to categorize health care resources is to think of them as directed primarily toward preventive care, acute care, and chronic care. Most localities of sufficient size provide a number of facilities and resources available to older persons for preventive health care. Among these are private physicians, dentists, and optometrists who give routine checkups and perform diagnostic checks. Many communities provide free or low-cost health clinics for routine health-screening procedures and immunizations. Increasingly, acute care hospitals are offering health education and screening programs for the well elderly. In a growing number of communities, health maintenance organizations (HMOs) are being developed. Usually involving physicians and a number of other health professionals, HMOs have prevention as a major goal. For a regular monthly fee, a wide variety of medical services is available from prevention to treatment and rehabilitation. When one joins an HMO, a comprehensive examination is often recommended at the outset to diagnose preexisting conditions and to plan a program of preventive care. HMO patients are encouraged to return as soon as they notice symptoms that bother them, rather than wait until they are certain something is wrong. The thinking behind HMOs is that if people have paid in advance for health care, they will be more likely to seek prompt attention. Problems will be detected and treated earlier, thus potentially reducing the need for further treatment and reducing the overall cost of health care.

Acute Care

Acute care refers to attention to a presumably short-term ailment that is already manifesting itself. Most older persons consult their family physician or internist when they believe they need acute medical care, but some do not have a personal physician. If the problem requires prompt attention (particularly during the night or weekends), they often seek help at a hospital emergency room or trauma center. Unless the problem appears to be one that is life threatening or will require hospital admission, this can be an inappropriate use of health care resources. Generally trauma centers are designed to provide prompt help for persons with serious, immediate problems (for example, heart attack, respiratory failure, stroke) and are expensive places to treat less severe problems. In response to this, immediate care centers have been developed in a number of communities. Staffed days, nights, and weekends by a group of physicians, these centers are designed to give prompt attention to acute problems of persons who do not have personal physicians or whose physicians are not available at the time the problem occurs.

Many older persons spend time in acute care hospitals when they have major surgery or suffer from illnesses that cannot be easily treated at home. In response to the high cost of hospital care, physicians are now required to discharge their patients earlier from hospitals than was previously the case. Lower cost convalescent centers are available in some localities for those whose care following surgery or an illness requiring hospitalization cannot be managed at home. Home health services (for example, nurses, physical therapists, speech therapists) are available to those recovering from an acute problem, usually at lower cost than an extended hospital stay.

Not long ago, nearly all surgery was done in acute care hospitals, with the patient remaining in the hospital for post-operative recovery and observation. Now some types of surgery are performed in one-day surgical units of hospitals or in free-standing surgical centers. Patients typically have surgery in the morning and are discharged to their homes by the end of the day. Surgery for cataracts and hernias may be performed in these units if no complications are anticipated.

Health Care for Chronic Conditions

As noted earlier, most older persons with chronic conditions live in their own homes and experience few major limitations on their daily activities. They usually consult frequently with their physicians about their conditions and may travel to receive specialized treatment (for example, physical therapy or speech therapy).

For persons whose chronic problems limit their mobility, home health services may be prescribed. Under the supervision of a physician, a nurse will visit with the patient in his or her own home, provide needed treatments, and report to the physician on the patient's condition. Speech therapy and physical therapy may also be provided at home, as may personal care services, which include help with bathing, grooming, and preparation of meals. Home health care is an important aspect of long-term care.

For a variety of reasons, some older persons with chronic conditions cannot be cared for at home, and their problems are not of the kind dealt with in acute care hospitals. Such persons are typically referred to nursing homes, residential facilities that provide around-the-clock nursing supervision and custodial care. Nursing home care is controversial and is dealt with at length in Chapter 12. We mention nursing homes at this point since they are the most prominent facilities providing care for the chronically ill elderly.

Earlier we noted that some older persons suffer from cancer from which they are expected to die within a relatively short period of time. Some with incurable cancer and other fatal illnesses prefer to receive treatment aimed at their comfort rather than the extension of their lives. Within the last ten years or so, many communities have developed hospice organizations to help such patients and their families live as comfortably as possible with the illness and impending death. Most hospice organizations offer home care, focused on relieving pain—physical, psychological, and social. Visiting nurses, aides, social workers, clergy, dietitians, and nonprofessional volunteers provide education, professional services, and support. Medication is prescribed to hospice patients with the goal of keeping them as pain-free and alert as possible. Some hospice programs provide inpatient facilities for acute care the family cannot provide at home, but inpatient stays are generally expected to be brief. Overall, the hospice philosophy is to help the patient live out his or her life as comfortably as possible in a familiar environment with a minimum of intrusive medical procedures.

Paying for Health Care Services

Health care is costly, and as noted earlier, older persons are disproportionately high consumers of health care services. The American Association of Retired Persons (1985) reports what while those sixty-five and older represented 12 percent of the U.S. population in 1984, they accounted for 31 percent of the nation's personal health care expenditures. Further, the average yearly medical bill for older persons was approximately $4,302. Thanks to a number of government and private health insurance programs available to older persons, most do not pay the full cost of their health care out of their own pockets. Nevertheless, older persons, on the average, pay about one-fourth of their health care bills from their own resources, with the remainder coming primarily from the various types of insurance programs available to them. In this section, we discuss a variety of programs available to help older persons with their health care bills.

Medicare

Since 1965, the federal government has assisted older persons in meeting their health care bills through the Medicare program. Financed through taxes paid by workers covered by Social Security and by premiums paid by older beneficiaries, Medicare pays about half of the total elderly health care bills (U.S. Senate Special Committee on Aging, 1985).

Persons eligible for OASDHI benefits apply for Medicare coverage when they apply for retirement or disability benefits. Medicare hospital insurance (Part A) includes benefits for inpatient hospital care, medically necessary care in a skilled nursing facility following a hospital stay, home health care, and hospice care. Legislation passed in October 1988 will require the patient to pay a deductible estimated to be around $565 for 1989. Unlike the previous plan, which had a co-insurance feature, the new plan pays all covered hospital costs beyond the deductible. Allowances for skilled nursing home care, home health care, and hospice care have all been increased.

Most medical facilities accept Medicare hospital insurance and bill Medicare directly. The beneficiary must pay the deductible and charges for any services not covered by the program, such as private duty nurses or custodial care (known as intermediate care) in nursing homes. The Part A benefits are financed by a portion of the payroll tax paid by each employer and employee or by each self-employed person.

Persons eligible for hospital insurance may choose to purchase Medicare medical insurance (Part B). The monthly premium ($24.80 in 1988) is deducted from their Social Security checks. Beginning in 1989, a patient's liability is limited to a payment of the first $75 and 80 percent of any remaining covered charges, up to a limit of $1,370 for any year. Covered charges include physicians' services, diagnostic tests, medical supplies, special therapies (physical and speech), and a number of outpatient hospital services.

These new features for Part B are financed by an additional premium of $4.00 a month and a supplemental premium based on one's federal income tax liability. Beginning in 1990, Medicare will pay some drug costs. By 1993, Medicare will cover 80 percent of a patient's drug costs above $710 per year. Previously, the cost of self-administered drugs was not covered. For more complete information, consult the latest edition of *Your Medicare Handbook*, available at any Social Security office.

There are a number of medical services not covered by Medicare that are very important to good health in later life. These include routine physical examinations, routine foot care, eyeglasses and hearing aids and services to prescribe and fit them, most immunizations, and most dental services and dentures.

While very important in reducing the out-of-pocket health care costs of older persons, having Medicare by no means fully insures older persons against the costs of health services. For some, coming up with the initial deductible for a hospital stay or visit to a physician represents a barrier to seeking health care early. Older persons on limited budgets are often frustrated by Medicare payment mechanisms. Many physicians and other health care providers expect patients to pay the full cost of service at the time it is provided. It is then up to the patient to submit a claim for Medicare reimbursement.

Submitting a claim can be a bewildering experience. Claim forms appear complicated, particularly to persons with limited education. While they expect reimbursement for some of the bill they have already paid, they cannot be sure how much the reimbursement will be or when it will arrive. For those without substantial financial reserves, this can create a cash flow problem, resulting in financial hardship.

In view of the number of things for which Medicare does not pay or pays limited amounts, it is not surprising that older persons who can afford it typically purchase supplementary medical insurance. Sometimes, retired persons are able to continue with a group policy offered by their former employer if they pay the premium themselves. Others purchase supplemental health insurance from companies with which they had no previous association. Generically known as "medigap insurance," supplemental health insurance policies vary widely in costs and coverage. The consumer is well advised to shop carefully for a good policy.

Medicaid

Older persons classified as poor may be eligible for assistance with their health care bills through the Medicaid program in their state. Medicaid is financed by a combination of federal and state tax revenues and administered by state agencies. Provisions vary widely from state to state. Generally, Medicaid coverage is much more extensive than Medicare coverage. Most Medicaid programs, for example, pay for custodial care in nursing homes. In some states, more extensive home health benefits than those offered by Medicare are available. Through arrangements with Medicare, Medicaid pays poor older persons' premiums for medical insurance, making them eligible for coverage available to Medicare patients. Since eligibility criteria and services covered vary under the Medicaid program, readers are encouraged to consult with their local or state Medicaid office for details about how Medicaid can help persons with whom they work.

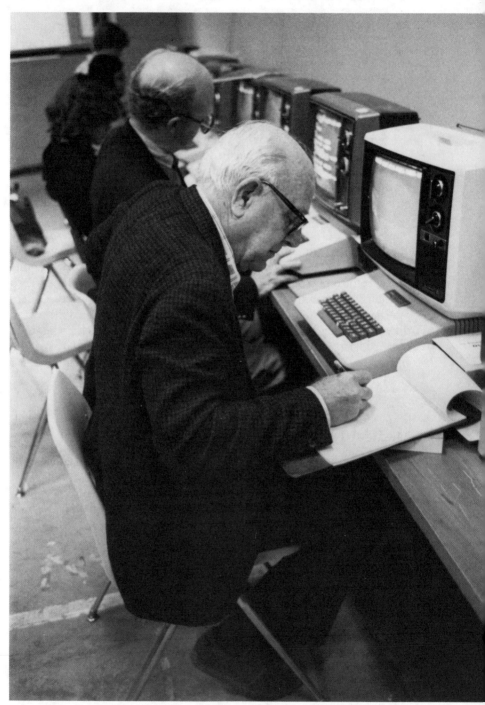

5

Mental Health

There is a persistent myth about older people that has become firmly entrenched in popular culture. In novels and on television, older people are frequently portrayed as senile, forgetful, helpless old crocks who create problems for the younger generation. Recently, one of the authors saw a bumper sticker that said, "Get even—live long enough to be a problem to your children!" While there are older people who do suffer from mental health problems, this is not true of the majority of aged persons. Most older persons are perfectly capable of managing their affairs. In fact, many older people remain creative and active well into their eighties and nineties.

Pablo Casals, the famous cellist, was performing well up into his nineties. George Washington Carver was still discovering uses for the peanut and the soybean in his seventies. Leonardo da Vinci was active until he was quite old. Ruth Gordon, the award-winning actress and playwright, had a career that lasted over fifty years. These well-known people are not exceptions. Many "ordinary" older people are mentally healthy. Good mental health in old age is the norm rather than the exception.

Why, then, all the concern with senility, forgetfulness, and incompetence? It is the old story of the dramatic cases overshadowing the usual. The older person who has a mental or emotional disorder *is* a problem to himself or herself and to the family. The sharp-minded older person is not a problem, and thus goes virtually unnoticed by the casual observer.

What Is Satisfactory Mental Health?

Before we can talk about the mental health problems of the older person, it makes sense to come to some conclusion about what satisfactory mental health is. For too long, we have only looked at mental problems (and this is true at all ages) without paying proper attention to the state of health. We argue that mental health is not just the absence of disease, but instead is a state in which the person glows with health. While we cannot give a definition that will satisfy everybody, we will make plain what we consider a state of good mental health before we discuss those situations that are unhealthy.

We will draw on what may sound an unlikely source, since it comes from a text on childhood and adolescence. Doing so is not as incongruous as it may sound. If one is going to think intelligently about child development, one must have some notion about *development for what*. Some years ago, Joseph Stone and Joseph Church postulated the positive outcome of healthy child development. The following quotation states their basic position.

> It is our thesis that maturity . . . can and should be a time of fulfillment, of continued growth and repeated discoveries and insights, of ever-renewed enthusiasm, of fresh understanding and solid wisdom. One has a choice. He can spend maturity and old age looking wistfully back on the good old days or he can, more than at any other period, relish the joys of the moment, savor the zest of things, and look forward to the excitements of the future. He (or she) can keep physically fit and vigorous, or he can strive foolishly to preserve the powers of youth, or he can cave in and go to seed. (Stone and Church, 1973: 491)

Stone and Church go on to expand their definition of maturity, which we will follow closely in the next paragraphs. The reader should consult the original for the full discussion, but we will summarize it here for our present purpose (Stone and Church, 1973: 492–99).

The mentally healthy older person is one who is capable of continued change. Of course, this change is within some limits. One could not decide at seventy-five to become the starting quarterback for the Chicago Bears! However, one should be able to change, given what he or she has become in previous years. Healthy older persons are capable of self-determination to the extent that they should be able to accept or refuse choices from among those that are available. Some choices in old age will have been precluded by choices made earlier in life. As an example, Stone and Church point out that at the age of ninety, one could not choose to be a full-fledged member of another culture, even if one moved to another country. Such a person would always be a kind of "transplant" because his or her development had taken place elsewhere.

Old age is also a time when a person can cultivate wisdom. This is not, in Stone and Church's view, the tendency to pontificate, but the ability to display "insight, sensitivity, understanding, tolerance." One becomes emotionally stable in healthy old age, and is not driven by every wind of novelty. He or she can change, but can also maintain the integrity that has been developed up to this point. Mentally healthy older people are "alive with vigorous interests that make (them) interesting to be with."

The healthy older person has a sense of humor. We would add to Stone and Church's discussion the often-quoted advice that healthy people should never take things too seriously, starting with themselves! Healthy humor is not destructive of other persons, but it does see and appreciate those things that are genuinely funny.

The healthy older person is, say Stone and Church, "at home with reality." This does not mean that the older person is obliged to like everything, but it does mean that he or she has come to understand how things are and can work with reality as it is rather than as they would like it to be. The healthy person also is at home with himself. While this does not mean that healthy people think they are perfect, it does mean that they know their limitations and have come to accept the kind of people they are and can master their own feelings.

Healthy people set a high priority on worthwhile human relationships and they are concerned with important social problems. While they no longer believe that they can lick the world unaided, they will involve themselves in important things and they will take risks on behalf of important political and social issues.

Mentally healthy people also need solitude from time to time and they enjoy solitary activities. They do not accept values without question, but are thoughtful and selective about what they believe and what they consider important. Further, they are committed to the values they hold, and are willing to act on them. Although they may sometimes have unconventional attitudes, they respect the feelings of others and do not enter into disputes lightly.

Finally, healthy people are conscious of their mortality. This is not a source of discomfort, but adds to their appreciation of the importance of what they do. Since they know they will not live forever, they try to involve themselves in activities they think are worth doing and avoid worrying over trifles.

Although the longer statement that we have summarized here was written in the early 1970s, it is still valid, and for that matter, was valid in our grandparents' day. There is a kind of timelessness about the qualities of maturity and good mental health, and this view will still be useful one hundred years from now. It is very close to the definition of the self-actualizing person offered by A. H. Maslow (1954) over thirty years ago.

Few people exemplify all of these characteristics, but some exhibit a good many of them. Obviously, the closer people are to this pattern, the healthier they are and the less likely they will need interventive services. The point we want to make is that most older Americans do have a healthy maturity, and their mental health is extremely good. There is little that we need to do to serve these people. In fact, what we should do is to enlist them in our efforts to help those who have not been able to achieve emotional stability and a sense of mastery over life. Mature healthy people can provide a great deal of service as volunteers or as paid members of institutional or agency staff.

With this as background, we can now consider the difficulties that arise with the older person who does not have the social and emotional resources of the mentally healthy elderly.

Barriers to Satisfactory Mental Health

It is important to recognize that there are major sources of difficulty that threaten the state of satisfactory mental health. We will discuss these sources of difficulty under two broad headings: (1) factors in the social structure and (2) factors in the individual situation.

Structural Factors

We must admit that there is a certain amount of chance in successful aging, even though we believe that, in general, the larger part of the outcome of one's life is determined by the way in which one participates in life. Chance enters into those situations in which one has limited power to effect change, for example, when and where one is born, and the general conditions of the times. Even then, one's response to the circumstances of life is highly individual, and many people have been able to live exemplary lives even when the odds were heavily against them.

As noted in chapter 3, successful aging takes a certain amount of financial security. This does not mean that everyone who would be a mentally healthy older person needs to be wealthy. It does suggest that most people need enough money to provide adequate food, suitable shelter, clothing, and a decent level of medical care in order to sustain their healthy state.

Factors in the social system that interfere with one's ability to survive constitute one kind of threat to one's mental health. Consequently, those elements in a society that threaten one's basic existence constitute conditions that spawn mental and emotional problems. Some of these factors are clearly economic; others are more easily seen as broader societal factors that involve social mores, traditions, and politics.

Poverty

First, let us take up the question of poverty. We read in our newspapers that poverty among the elderly has declined in the 1980s to the point that only about 12 to 14 percent are defined as poor using the federal government's definition. This is lower than the rate of poverty in the society as a whole, and it is true as far as it goes. However, rather than rejoicing about the lowered level of poverty among the old, we need to think about the effect of being poor on those older persons who remain among the economically disadvantaged, including those who are just over the poverty line.

Poverty is complex, and this is not the place to digress into a lengthy discussion about either causes or effects. Here we want to focus on its consequences for mental and emotional health. We said earlier that one did not need to be wealthy to enjoy a financially secure old age. One does have to have enough. What is enough? That depends upon the lifestyle that one is willing to accept. We know people who live in remote rural areas who have very little. However, their mental health is good. Is it because they are too ignorant to know what they lack and therefore are unknowing victims of structural poverty? We think not. The people that we have in mind are content because they have enough to follow the pattern that they have worked out in their lives. But what about the people who have not been able to live as they could reasonably have expected? There are several consequences for their mental health that we need to consider.

In our consideration, we will not go into the general effect of poverty on health. Obviously, people without enough to live on will develop serious health problems including those conditions related to vitamin deficiencies, dental problems, digestive system disorders, and the host of other illnesses related to bad diet. In this discussion, we will confine ourselves to the effect that poverty has on one's emotional stability and general outlook on life.

As one would suspect, poverty generally has a psychologically depressing effect on most people. Only a few saints rejoice in being poor, but they have chosen to be poor, and the effects of poverty are negated by their joy in service to their cause. For those who are not saints, however, there is little joy in being unable to afford to have a decent level of existence.

We are not talking now of clinical depression. We will take that up later. What we want to discuss here is the general overall level of discomfort that occurs among otherwise healthy people who simply cannot live a life that is satisfactory to them. While the short-run consequences are minimal and reversible, over the long run, chronically poor people acquire a persistent sense of depression that may be subclinical but is nevertheless a source of genuine discomfort. This effect is stubborn, and cannot simply be "therapized" away because it often has its source largely outside the individual's control. As an example, consider a man who has been employed over the greater part of his life at a moderately well-paying job in the auto industry. Suppose this man is laid off at age sixty. He will be eligible for unemployment compensation for at least twenty-six weeks, and maybe longer, depending on the state in which he lives. If this man is not called back to work he will be forced to get by as best he can until he becomes eligible for early retirement at sixty-two. In twenty years time, we could very well find this man chronically depressed solely because of his poor economic position.

Although this is a hypothetical example, it is not far from reality for many people. The situation is worse for many women who are now in their seventies and eighties. Many women remained in the home in previous years and held no income-producing job. Consequently, they receive no OASDHI payments beyond what they receive as wives of retired workers. They will continue to receive benefits if they survive their spouses, but these benefits are reduced from the total that the couple would have received. It is no wonder that these people live in a chronic state of "the blues" even though the depression may not be severe enough to warrant full-scale psychiatric treatment.

Retirement

Traditionally, retirement was viewed as a negative event for many people. Before World War II, only two kinds of people retired: those who had a lot of money and could retire comfortably, and those who had no choice in the matter but were retired because of bad health or because the organization simply considered them too old. This narrow view of retirement no longer prevails. Today, large numbers of people retire at sixty-five or even earlier if they can afford to do so (as we saw in chapter 3). Retirement is no longer seen as an automatic consignment to the rubbish heap. Atchley (1985) has extensively reviewed the literature on retirement and he reports that if one is satisfied with his or her life, retirement is a healthy state of being. Whether one is satisfied has to do with the state of one's health, income, accomplishments, the family, and other personal factors. Atchley found no study that suggests that retirement automatically has a negative effect on one's mental health. Mental health problems may *cause* some to retire, but it rarely is the other way around. Atchley does note that those who are better off financially, better educated, and who have been employed at higher-status jobs do have more positive views of retirement than those who are poor, badly educated, and have held low-status jobs. He also notes that older people, in general, do not become socially isolated, nor do they disengage themselves from activities that are satisfying.

Retirement, then, is a traumatic event for only limited numbers of older people. Generally, we can say that for those who do not have a sense of accomplishment with their working careers, whose health is bad, and who lack money, the adjustment to retirement can be emotionally difficult. Currently, because economic conditions have been good for the middle- and upper-income segments of the population, a large number of people (around 40 percent) choose early retirement. The operative word here is *choose*. There is a difference between what people choose for themselves and what is forced on them by policy. For those older persons who experience the job as their whole life and for whom there are no obvious alternatives, retirement will likely be the most difficult.

Geographical location

Another structural factor that can affect the mental and emotional health of older persons has to do with where they live. Again, we must stress that the bulk of older people live in houses that are in satisfactory repair or in apartments that provide adequate comfort. However, this is not universal. Large numbers of older people live in houses in need of repair, cheap apartments, or decaying retirement hotels. Often these less satisfactory homes are in older neighborhoods that in effect become ghettos of frightened, anxious older people who are victimized by the hustlers and human jackals that live in any society. Of course, part of the problem relates to the economic difficulties that we mentioned earlier. Part of it, however, simply has to do with the structural position of older people in a society that values youth. Age is no protection against thieves, rapists, and burglars. People who live in enclaves of poverty spend a great deal of time simply trying to protect what little they have and survive as best they can. Because of their limited income, they cannot afford the elaborate security of the more affluent. Many cannot afford the cost of deadbolts and burglar-proof locks on windows. There is little protection on the street, and many elders are afraid to go out after dark. One of the authors knows of a situation in which an older man confined to a wheelchair and living alone was robbed repeatedly by the same group of youths. They turned off the lights when they entered his house and often greeted him familiarly by telling him, "Pops, we're back again!"

Older people in these neighborhoods repeatedly have Social Security and Supplemental Security Income checks stolen from their mailboxes. Although direct deposit of these checks is possible, many older people like to see the check and do not take advantage of the government's offer to send the check directly to a bank. As a holdover from the Great Depression when many banks failed, some older persons do not trust banks.

While the kind of daily fear that is experienced by older people who live in unsafe neighborhoods is usually not enough to cause severe emotional problems, it certainly adds to the other burdens that they carry. Further, because the neighborhood is the way it is, these older people may find it difficult to locate sources of help.

Many of these neighborhoods are close to the decayed central portions of the city. We know of several communities—including the city in which the authors live—where there are no grocery stores within walking distance of a significant number of older people. Even a trip to the Social Security office is difficult, unless one is able to drive or has a friend with a car. Public transportation is unavailable in many medium and small cities, and is unsafe in many of the larger ones. Because poor older people are not perceived as politically powerful, there is little concern on the part of elected officials; they do not act in ways that can be helpful unless forced to do so. Consequently, the older person, trapped in decaying age-segregated neighborhoods, adds a feeling of powerlessness to his or her growing burden of problems. This increases the daily anxiety under which the older person must live.

Sex discrimination and racism

There are two other social structural factors that can contribute to problems in the emotional health of older people. First, there is no doubt that women have suffered from persistent and not very subtle discrimination. This discrimination has had particularly deleterious effects for older women. Perhaps, as the economic and social status of women changes over time, many of the effects of discrimination will pass. Until that time, those who are in service occupations will continue to encounter emotional problems related to discrimination.

Earlier, we noted that older women are publicly perceived as less interesting and less desirable as partners than younger women. To the extent that this social attitude affects an individual woman, it constitutes a source of anxiety for her. Older women may also find that they are taken less seriously by a variety of service providers unless they have money and status. This is probably most crucial when the service provider is the older woman's physician. Unfortunately, some physicians still do not listen to the complaints of the older woman, and see her symptoms as imaginary when they may be indicative of a serious illness.

In general, the relative powerlessness of women in our society is exacerbated in old age. The lower income relative to men, the generally lower status of women's occupations, and the degree to which women have experienced discrimination in social and business relationships are factors that service providers need to be aware of for their possible effects on the emotional health of a given woman.

The discussion above can be extended to cover the effect of racism on those older persons of color in society. While many individuals have been able to surmount the barriers of racism and carve out successful lives that provide them with the prerequisites for successful aging, many continue to suffer from oppression. While structural or institutional racism is a lifelong source of difficulty, it has an especially poignant effect on the aged. Like women, older people of color bring to old age the accumulated effects of past discrimination. Those who work with elderly members of racial and cultural minorities must be aware of the possibility that discrimination may have contributed to the psychosocial difficulties that a given person experiences.

Ageism

The generalized attitude that finds its expression in a set of stereotyped and negative evaluations of older people has become known as ageism. Ageism is related to many elements of the structural problems that we have identified above. Despite our increase in knowledge about aging, there is still a persistent belief that the aged are less capable—and less important—than other people. Ageism can be a barrier to obtaining quality services. If service providers believe that the aged are less valuable than other members of society, they may render a lower quality of service. Beyond that, older people are well aware of the way others feel, so that the fact of ageism's existence has a negative effect on the mental and emotional health of older people.

Individual Factors

Beyond the structural factors summarized above, there are other things that relate primarily to the individuals involved. Dr. R. N. Butler, former director of the National Institute on Aging, and M. E. Lewis, a social worker, have listed a number of factors (including some of the structural problems that we have discussed earlier) that they classify as age-related emotional factors affecting the mental health of older people (Butler and Lewis, 1982). We will follow Butler and Lewis' lead in discussing these factors, but we have interspersed a number of comments and examples for which Butler and Lewis are not responsible. Actually, these problems can occur at any age (and do), but they are more likely, by their nature, to occur as we grow older. Some of the problems discussed below will need to be referred to a specialized agency or institution, so we will review some principles of referral at the end of the chapter.

Age-Related Emotional Factors

First, there is the problem that occurs when one loses a spouse through death. This often is a psychologically devastating event. In modern industrial cultures, the problem is compounded by the tendency to deny the reality of death and the decline of commonly understood mourning rituals. In previous centuries, death took place in the home and the dying person, along with the people that he or she left behind, had more control over the dying process. The immediate community shared the family's grief and entered actively into everyday supportive behavior.

Today, death usually takes place in institutions where the fact of death is concealed or downplayed as much as possible. For example, some hospitals have carts with false bottoms that permit the movement of bodies in the hospital while the cart appears empty.

The family is often scattered, and the sense of community is often absent because of the larger size of modern cities. Universally recognizable mourning customs, even symbolic gestures, such as widow's veils and widower's mourning bands (a black cloth band worn on the sleeve) have disappeared, and one is encouraged to "get back to normal" as soon as possible.

Grief at the loss of a loved one is a perfectly natural phenomenon, and we are less than human when we pass off a loss of major magnitude as if it were a minor inconvenience. Clinically, a mourning period of two to three years is within normal limits. It is common, in fact, for grief symptoms to recur for many years, especially on the birthday of the deceased or on significant holidays. Typically, one experiences one or more of a number of symptoms. It is not unusual to experience disturbed sleep patterns, a loss of appetite, and difficulties in the digestive system with a consequent loss of weight. One also has persistent feelings of sadness and loss. At the thought of the deceased, one may even experience choking sensations and breathlessness. Anxiety, guilt, and a sense of inner tension may also be present.

Some writers see grief as a stage process. DeSpelder and Strickland (1987: 212–17) have reviewed the major theories of grief. While the theories differ in detail, they generally agree that grief begins with a period of shock and disbelief, followed by one or more stages of pain and emotional upheaval. Eventually, one regains his or her balance. When grief symptoms persist to the point at which the survivor's ability to get on with the business of living is seriously affected, they constitute a chronic grief reaction. At that point, intervention should be considered seriously. In chapter 9, some of the major issues in working with a surviving spouse are discussed and illustrated in the case of the Benson family.

In addition to normal grief, some survivors may defend themselves against the shock of losing a spouse by extreme denial. They attempt to carry on as if the deceased spouse were still living and will come home any time. The authors know of instances in which the surviving spouses have kept the deceased spouses' clothes cleaned and pressed and hanging in closets for many years. These situations are often difficult to deal with and they usually require medical intervention. Persons who deliver services to older persons should be alert to these situations and be prepared to assist the older person and his or her family to approach a specialized resource that can help.

Another age-related problem noted by Butler and Lewis is marital difficulty. Many couples find themselves thrown together more in old age and they sometimes discover that they no longer like each other very much. Often these are couples who have raised a family. As a rule, couples without children have already either become securely interdependent, or have parted company long before they grew old.

When the children have grown and gone off on their own, many of the shared tasks and concerns that were part of the marital bond become irrelevant.

In the popular literature, this is often referred to as the empty nest syndrome, an oversimplication of a much more complicated situation. Most couples enjoy the freedom that ensues when children become adults. Further, they find that the new adult relationships they have with their children are more satisfying and enjoyable than the former ones. Recently, the authors heard the expression, "Life begins when the last child leaves the house and the old dog dies!" The implication is that much of the routine of family life can now be exchanged for a freer existence.

However, the joy that many experience is not universal. While it is hard to generalize, it is fair to say that the marriages that had underlying difficulties during earlier stages are the ones most likely to develop serious problems in old age. Although routines and tasks of family life may have kept the problems submerged for a time, the couple did not really resolve them. Now, with the children gone and on their own, the couple is left with the problems and few or none of the tasks that permitted the problems to be sublimated or repressed. Of course, it may be possible for the couple to find new ways to avoid confronting their difficulties. The partners may each develop new interests that permit them to invest themselves in activity that avoids the problems. They may become emotionally separate, even though they continue to share the same house.

In some cases, this kind of avoidance actually works well. However, in many situations it does not. With the luxury of time at their disposal, the couple may turn on each other and a lifetime of hurt and disappointment may surface to threaten the relationship. Here again, couples with severe marital difficulty should be offered the opportunity for marital counseling. We know of no communities with counseling agencies solely devoted to working with the older couple. Most communities, however, do have some form of family counseling agency that can be of help.

Another crisis occurs when one of the pair becomes ill, and the other has to assume the role of nurse. This role may create a number of strains that sorely test the unity of the couple. Again, the underlying health of the relationship is an important factor. Couples that have functioned well before usually continue to function well when one partner becomes ill. Couples with a great deal of pathology in their relationship often find that the serious illness of one partner brings it to the surface. For example, some years ago, one of the authors had a friend who was dying of cancer. When he visited the friend, all the friend's spouse could talk about was the expense and inconvenience of her husband's illness. While this attitude might be regarded as a defense against painful reality, the author's conclusion was that it was a genuine reflection of long-held feelings that the husband had always been an inconvenience. The illness had merely worsened the underlying dissatisfaction with the marriage.

Butler and Lewis observe that sexual problems sometimes arise in older years when they didn't occur before. Usually these are related to illness (the difficulty of intercourse when one partner is wearing a colostomy bag), but they may relate to boredom or the (usually unwarranted) fear of a coronary.

Finally, Butler and Lewis record the potentially damaging effect of increasing illnesses, including sensory loss (deafness, loss of acute sight), and the effects of pain from chronic diseases as in the case of arthritis. They claim that 86 percent of older persons have some kind of chronic health problem (some of which are slight, but others of which are serious) that may constitute threats to one's emotional health. Any one of these health problems may include psychological symptoms that complicate the original illness.

In addition to the above, Butler and Lewis list a number of emotional reactions: guilt, loneliness, mild depression, anxiety (about health, money), sense of helplessness, and rage at life. All these reactions seem to reflect the loss of meaning in life that some disappointed older people experience when things have not turned out as they had hoped.

While the above factors are widely recognized, Butler and Lewis add another that is of unusual interest. They suggest that it is natural for one to engage in a "life review" as one grows older. They see this as a natural process in which one reassesses his or her life and is either depressed or satisfied, depending on how things add up. For those for whom life has not turned out too badly, the life review can be therapeutic. However, Butler and Lewis note that "the most tragic life review is that in which a person decides life was a total waste" (Butler and Lewis, 1982, p. 59). It is this kind of person who often commits suicide. While we think that these suicides can be forestalled in the short run, if these people cannot find something worthwhile in their lives, they are in danger in the long run.

With the exception of suicide, the problems listed above are manageable with a moderate amount of intervention. However, we will now turn to some disorders that probably will require more intensive help. These are serious mental and emotional disorders that can be subsumed under two major headings: functional disorders and organic brain disorders.

Serious Mental and Emotional Disorders

Some preliminary remarks are in order. First, it must be said that the kind of mental and emotional disorders seen in older people are not radically different from the disorders seen in younger people. Butler and Lewis state flatly that "Older persons . . . have the same psychiatric disorders as the young with similar genesis and structure." We have been so brainwashed by popular fiction and slick journalism that we have come to believe that the diseases of old age are of a different order than those of earlier life. This simply is not so. While there may be a higher occurrence of some of these disorders in old age, they are the same disorders.

Butler and Lewis make two other important points. First, it is more important to assess the *functioning* of older people than simply to arrive at a diagnosis. There are people with relatively serious illnesses who function fairly well because they have good support from those around them. There are others who are less ill but more in need of assistance because they lack familial and social support. Second, a psychiatric diagnosis may not mean a lot, simply because physicians often try to protect their patients from the consequences of more serious diagnoses for employment and insurance purposes. As an example, some years ago one of the authors was in training in a large teaching hospital. He got on the elevator with a surgeon and a psychiatrist. Observing that the author was wearing the customary white coat of the hospital employee, the doctors were less closemouthed than they otherwise might have been. The surgeon was berating the psychiatrist, whom he had called in for a consultation. "Why did you give my patient that diagnosis?"

"Well, what did you want me to do?" replied the psychiatrist.

"I didn't want you to give him that diagnosis. He'll never work again with that on his medical record," said the surgeon.

"So what can I do now?" the psychiatrist asked.

"You can go back up there and change the diagnosis. Can't you call it a situational reaction?" insisted the surgeon.

As the author left the elevator, the surgeon charged past him toward the coffee shop, while the psychiatrist, frowning, pressed the "up" button on the elevator and headed back upstairs, presumably to change the diagnosis to something less damaging.

We reproduce this conversation as a warning to those who work with patients. The moral is that one should observe the general ability of the individual to function and avoid becoming enamored of the official diagnosis. It may be a matter of convenience, and not at all reflective of the person's actual functioning, which may be better or worse than the diagnosis would indicate.

Functional disorders

Mental health professionals generally divide serious mental problems into two broad categories: functional disorders (those believed to arise from the person's psychosocial situation) and organic disorders (those believed to have a physiological or organic cause). This distinction may not really be appropriate since some disorders traditionally labeled functional may be related to organic factors, and some that are considered organic have psychosocial components. We will take the traditional approach here because it remains in common use.

We will use the terminology found in the American Psychiatric Association's *Diagnostic and Statistical Manual of Mental Disorders*. The current edition (hereafter referred to as the *DSM-III-R*) was published in 1987. The terminology in the *DSM-III-R* is used to classify recognizable mental disorders for both clinical and research purposes. We will not go into an extensive description of the disorders that we will discuss; consult the *DSM-III-R* for details. Human service personnel should have a copy of the current *Diagnostic and Statistical Manual* available to be able to understand the terminology used in reports from consulting psychiatrists, clinical psychologists, and mental health facilities. A new edition will be available after 1992.

While we have stressed that most older persons are mentally healthy, people who work with older people should be aware of symptoms that are potentially serious and deserve attention. Some of these symptoms come on suddenly, while others are more insidious in their development. Often these symptoms may be attributed to "old age" and thus are not recognized as symptoms of serious disease. In fact, none of these symptoms is the result of aging as such. Although they occur more frequently in older people, they occur in persons of any age. When they are seen in younger people, they are more often regarded as symptoms of a disorder and are more likely to receive attention. The last point is a further example of the influence of societal discrimination toward the aging.

Mood disorders. Disorders in this classification, as one would expect, affect the person's mood. The most common symptom that should concern those who work with older people is often described as a serious case of the blues. The individual's demeanor is one of profound sadness. He or she may suffer from fatigue, loss of appetite with a resulting weight loss, and may talk of suicide. These symptoms may occur in persons with a serious disease (heart disease or cancer) or they may occur in otherwise apparently healthy people as the major aspect of the personality. Sometimes the person may alternate between episodes of depression and episodes of excessively active and unrealistic behavior (bi-polar disorder), but in older people one is most likely to see depression.

Those who work with older people should be concerned because these symptoms can be signs of a major depressive episode. Persons who are not qualified mental health professionals who work with the elderly should not decide who is seriously depressed and who is not. Always take seriously talk of suicide, and see to it that the older person who is chronically sad is seen by a qualified physician. Depression usually can be successfully treated by a combination of drugs and psychotherapy and may require a period of hospitalization. The grief that occurs when one is bereaved is not considered a mental disorder. However, prolonged grief may turn into a major depressive episode, so be aware of this when dealing with those who are bereaved.

Depression is generally considered to have its roots in an individual's personal situation unless it is clearly related to an organic disorder. An alternative school of thought suggests that chemical imbalances in the brain may cause depression, but since many depressions appear to be related to life crises, the chemical imbalance explanation has not been universally accepted.

Schizophrenia. Schizophrenia is a serious disorder that manifests itself primarily in a decline in ability to function in relationships with other people and with the real world. Bizarre delusions will often be present. The individual will flit from one unrelated thought to another, and may hear voices or have other hallucinations. There is often a lack of animation in people suffering from schizophrenia, and they often believe that they are controlled by outside forces. Most people think of the phrase "split personality" when they hear the word *schizophrenia,* which suggests a person who has two or more separate personalities. Actually, the word *split* refers to the increasing separation between reality and fantasy. Persons with this disorder exhibit an inability to distinguish between the real world as most people know it and some other reality known only to the sufferer.

As a general rule (and there are exceptions) schizophrenia is most likely to begin in the second or third decade of life. Some authorities believe that when schizophrenia occurs in older people, it is actually a recurrence of the disorder, which originated earlier in life.

The condition tends to come on very slowly. Many become chronic sufferers and gradually become less and less realistic. But it is not unusual for these persons to have long periods of remission when they are quite rational. Request a medical evaluation for those whose thinking gradually becomes muddled or confused and who exhibit delusions or hallucinations. These symptoms could mean schizophrenia or another of the serious conditions discussed below.

Delusional disorder. The *DSM-III-R* has replaced the term *paranoid disorder* with this term because the major characteristic of this disorder is delusion. There are a number of delusionary themes involved. The person may believe him- or herself loved by some public figure and may act out fantasies connected with that person. Or the individual may believe that he or she is a person of merit who has been overlooked by the world. Some victims suffer from an unjustified jealousy. Others believe themselves to be persecuted by one or more persons and may take violent action against those whom they perceive as persecutors. Still others believe that they have a bizarre and unwarranted physical disorder or disfigurement.

These symptoms may occur either as a major entity or as a complicating factor in other illnesses. Commonly, the person has an unfounded sense of persecution and thinks that "they (or some specific person) are out to get me." It must be recognized that this condition is properly seen as a symptom of delusional disorder only when there is no basis in reality for suspicion. It is a sad fact of life that many people have a well-founded sense of outside threat. When the threat is real, as may be the case in groups that suffer from discrimination, the sense of persecution is not a mental disorder. Many older people who live in dangerous neighborhoods have a justified fear for their lives.

It is not uncommon for an older person with a severe hearing loss to exhibit paranoid symptoms. They may believe that others are talking about them or looking at them unnecessarily. While this can and does occur in younger people with hearing loss, it is more common in older people whose hearing loss has persisted over time and grown worse. People who are geographically or emotionally isolated from significant others also may develop unrealistic suspicions that may border on delusions. Again, a qualified mental health professional should be consulted when an older person exhibits what may be delusionary thinking.

Hypochondriasis. This is a category with a number of somatoform disorders—physical symptoms that do not have organic or physiological cause. It is common in older people. Hypochondriacs are people who believe themselves seriously ill when there is no evidence for their belief. Many older people have health problems that are very serious, and they justifiably worry about them. Sometimes they become highly preoccupied with their bodily functions, but this is not true hypochondria. The distinction between genuine hypochondria and a morbid preoccupation with an organic condition may make little difference to the ill persons and those around them; life is uncomfortable in either case. Further, hypochondriacs eventually develop illnesses that have organic causes, so those who work with older people must take their complaints seriously and should refer the sufferer to his or her physician. In those who are not hypochondriacs, excessive body monitoring and talk of symptoms should be regarded as a cry for help, and appropriate therapeutic intervention should be sought.

Organic mental syndromes and disorders

Included here are disorders that have mental or emotional symptoms believed to be related to physiological or organic processes. Intelligence usually is not affected by age until very late in life. Scores on intelligence tests tend to rise into one's twenties and then level off and remain fairly constant. Therefore, when an older person exhibits a serious change in his or her ability to think, it is a sign of a serious problem. Some older people may become foggy and unaware of their surroundings. They may develop a poor short-term memory that goes beyond simple absent-mindedness. The ability to reason and see connections between things that are logically related may also decline. Often, their attention wanders, and they seem preoccupied with a subject that is not understandable to observers. They may lose control of their impulses and behave in ways that are uncharacteristic. A woman who has always been conservative about her appearance may dress in an extreme way. A man who has been well-spoken all his life may swear and engage in sexually explicit conversation. Members of either gender may engage in uncharacteristic sexually provocative behavior. They may also become irritable and excessively emotional, or unusually jittery and continually pick at objects or clothing. They may even have hallucinations and delusions. They may have severe sleep disturbances—persistently drowsy or wide awake for long periods of time. Any of these symptoms can occur alone or in combination with one or more others.

While some of these behaviors might concern us in a person of any age, they are especially important when they are uncharacteristic of an older person's ordinary behavior. We want to emphasize that we are not talking about eccentricities or ways of thinking or behavior that merely represent variations in a person's character. There are many people who do not think clearly—and never did. Many people are normally absent-minded and cannot remember where they put things or what they ate yesterday. We all know people who wander around in a fog for most of their lives. There is nothing necessarily wrong with adopting a new fashion either. Many older people characteristically adopt whatever is "in" even if it looks unbecoming, but these people were trendy when they were young. Many older persons have a healthy—or unhealthy—interest in sex that they have carried with them into old age. Older people do not sleep as much as they once did, nor are their sleep patterns what they used to be, so an occasional sleepless night should not be of concern. The major problem, as we see it, is that ageism may influence one's view of older people, leading one to see symptoms when they do not exist, or to ignore symptoms when they are indeed present.

The important thing is that when a way of thinking, feeling, or behaving differs markedly from one's characteristic pattern, it ought to be a matter of concern. These uncharacteristic behaviors may be signs of serious disorders that could be related to organic or physiological problems.

The writers of the *DSM-III-R* use the general term *organic mental syndrome* to describe mental difficulties that present a "constellation of psychological or behavioral signs and symptoms without reference to etiology" (DSM-III-R, 1987, p. 97). The term *organic mental disorder* is reserved for "a particular organic mental syndrome in which the etiology is known or presumed." Both terms refer to the same set of symptoms. An organic mental disorder is an organic mental syndrome for which a definite agent is considered responsible. Generally, when a person displays one of the groups of symptoms that comprise a syndrome, he or she will be diagnosed by the physician as having an *organic mental disorder* when the symptoms can be related to an illness (for example, an infection elsewhere in the body) or the effect of some toxic substance (for example, alcohol or withdrawal from alcohol). The most common organic mental syndromes in the aged are delirium, dementia, and intoxication and withdrawal.

Delirium. Delirium is primarily a state in which the individual appears to be in a fog. He or she has trouble paying attention to things going on in the surrounding environment. The person is confused and may have hallucinations, and his or her attention wanders. Generally, these symptoms come on suddenly in a matter of days or even hours.

While delirium can be related to a blow on the head, it is more likely caused by an infection outside the brain, disorders in metabolism, thiamine deficiency, kidney disease, the toxic effect of some ingested substance, or withdrawal from a substance (*DSM-III-R*, p. 102). Often, the symptoms will disappear if the underlying cause is successfully treated. If untreated, or if treatment is unsuccessful, the person may die.

Dementia. Dementia, on the other hand, does not present the fogginess of delirium. The most noticeable symptom is a memory loss. This may be something that occurs over a long period of time: it may be mild, or it may be so severe that the individual forgets his or her name and place of residence. The sufferer may cause harm to self or others by tinkering with some dangerous appliance. Even the simple act of making a cup of tea may present problems, since one suffering from dementia may put the kettle on and forget about it, resulting in a fire. As the memory deteriorates, so do personal standards of dress and cleanliness. The worst side of the personality emerges, and people who once seemed pleasant enough often develop frightening behaviors and damaging ways of relating to others. Over time, these people become increasingly withdrawn and remote. Eventually, they sink into a helpless state. The average life expectancy after the onset of symptoms is about five years, although some live ten or more years after onset.

The most common dementia is referred to in *DSM-III-R* as primary degenerative dementia of the Alzheimer type. Alzheimer's disease is not a mental disorder as such. It is a physical disease that has mental symptoms. Hence the reference to dementia of the Alzheimer type. A distinction is made between senile onset (after age sixty-five) and presenile onset (age sixty-five or below). The writers of *DSM-III-R* admit that this is an arbitrary distinction.

It has become popular to think that all dementia is related to Alzheimer's disease. There are, in fact, several other causes. *Multi-infarct dementia* is believed to be related to cerebrovascular disease. Over time, the person declines, but does so in steps. Some mental functions continue unaffected while others fail because the damage to the brain occurs in specific areas, or "patches." Other causes of dementia include central nervous system infections (which, in the aged, are more likely to include syphilis and tuberculosis than meningitis, viral encephalitis, and AIDS), head trauma, reactions to toxic substances, diet deficiencies, and various neurological diseases (including Huntington's chorea and Pick's disease). For the full list, consult *DSM-III-R* (p. 106).

Intoxication and withdrawal. Intoxication means something more than the effects of an occasional binge on some mind-altering substance. It involves the maladaptive behavior associated with the effect of the substance. Withdrawal symptoms include vomiting, irritability, and serious sleep problems, along with a craving for the substance that produced the intoxication.

Diagnosis of mental and neurological problems

Diagnosis is difficult even for the experts. Often the symptom picture is hard to sort out, and requires the use of sophisticated equipment. The worst danger is that an older person who is experiencing symptoms may be seen by family and friends as just "getting childish" in his or her old age and, therefore, may receive little or no treatment. It is important to refer the individual or his or her family to a qualified diagnostician.

First, the individual who works with older people who exhibit the serious symptoms discussed in this chapter needs to be alert to changes in mood, thinking, feelings, and behavior. One should not attribute changes to old age but should take seriously the deviations from the older person's characteristic mode of functioning.

Second, the helping person should focus on learning how to assist families in seeking help for relatives who exhibit these symptoms. We will discuss making referrals in general in chapter 11. However, since mental health problems usually represent a serious crisis for both the individual and his or her family, we want to give special attention to the mental health referral here.

1. Listen to the concerns of both the person to be referred and his or her family. It is difficult for people to face the possibility of serious mental illness, either in themselves or in those close to them. They need to be able to discuss these concerns in an accepting and positive atmosphere.
2. Do not give false reassurance by telling people that "things will be all right." *Do* assure the individual and the family that they are doing the proper thing by being concerned and seeking help.
3. Advise people of their options. This requires that the human service professional have a fairly sophisticated knowledge of the resources available.
4. Know the technical aspects of referral for any agency or institution to which you refer people. If you are going to refer a patient to X Memorial Hospital and Clinic, telephone or visit X Memorial before the conference in which the referral is made and find out what in-

formation, forms, or verifications are necessary. This is rarely done in practice. Often professionals say that they can't afford the time to pay "social calls" on agencies and institutions. We think that they can't afford *not* to. One in-person visit to a facility can help a professional avoid a lot of time-consuming memos and telephone calls about improper referrals.

5. Discuss, in general terms, what will likely happen at the place to which the referral is made (kinds of examinations or tests) with the patient and/or the family. This, too, can be learned through visits to various facilities. While the human service professional may not need to know all the details, he or she should be able to prepare the patient and family for the general procedure.

6. Provide the information that the agency or institution needs in a timely fashion. Veteran human service personnel have all been faced with the problem of clients or patients who have been referred to them with no accompanying request that explains the purpose of the referral. This wastes time for both the patient and the professional, who must then start from scratch.

7. Be in a position to advise the family on any fees or costs involved and any benefits to which they may be entitled. This may necessitate an additional referral to the welfare department, the Social Security office, or to a company personnel department so that an exact determination can be made.

8. Follow up. While we do not think that service professionals should harass people, it is good to make some contact with the patient or family, if for no other reason than to find out if some misunderstanding has occurred so that it can be corrected.

9. Be prepared to explain and interpret the diagnosis and proposed treatment after the family has completed the procedures at the agency or institution to which they have been referred. This will mean that the professional will need to maintain communications with the hospital, clinic, or other facility. Since this requires the permission of the family and/or patient, most agencies have forms that patients must sign to permit the exchange of information.

10. Again, listen for the patient's and family's concerns and respond supportively throughout the process.

A good referral doesn't just happen. It comes about when one is empathic to the family's concerns and frank in recognizing their fears and uncertainties. As a rule, the more concretely one can help people in these situations, the more effective the help will be.

6

Environmental Conditions

Regardless of age, one of the factors that influences our ability to carry out our activities successfully is the physical environment in which we find ourselves. When we are able to make choices about where we will live, we frequently take into account factors such as convenience, aesthetic value, safety, and access to resources. Characteristics of our private residences (apartments, houses, dorm rooms), of the space near our residences (corridors, halls, neighborhood), and of the communities in which we live can substantially affect our health and safety, our opportunities for social interactions, and our feelings of well-being. To take an obvious example, a person living in northern Minnesota in a home with a reliable source of home heating is likely to be healthier and safer than someone in the same environment without reliable heat. Similarly, persons who live in neighborhoods where street crime is a major problem risk social isolation and diminished feelings of well-being because they live in fear of being attacked.

In recent years, gerontologists have become increasingly interested in the relationships between characteristics of older persons' homes, neighborhoods, and communities and their physical and mental well-being. What is being learned can be of practical significance for persons who work for and on behalf of older persons. It is increasingly recognized that knowledge about the environment in which an older person lives can help us better understand his or her behavior. Accordingly, when professionals work with older persons, they frequently attempt to assess home environments, seeking the answers to questions including: Does the environment make it easier or more difficult for the older person to do what he or she wants to do? Are there features of the environment that might help us better understand problems the older person is experiencing? Can the environment be modified to accommodate to the older person's changing needs? Are there other living situations available that the older person might find more appropriate and more satisfying?

Professionals concerned with older persons may be called upon to make recommendations about location and design when housing for the aged is proposed. They may be asked for consultation on how to make existing institutions and planned communities for older persons more responsive to the residents' needs. Those working in the field of aging may also find themselves evaluating proposed neighborhood and community changes (for example, changes in zoning ordinances, the widening of a road) to determine what effect they are likely to have on older residents. They may be in a position to make recommendations about the type of housing for the aged that people want in a community or how neighborhoods could be changed to make them safer for older persons. Thus, whether the professional is working directly with older persons to improve their individual situations or is concerned about the well-being of older persons at a more global level, he or she can draw on knowledge about the interaction between aging and the physical environment in working to improve the lives of the aged.

This chapter has four major purposes. The first is to discuss a theoretical model that helps to account for the interactions between older persons and the demands of their physical environments. Second, we discuss how helping professionals can assist older persons who wish to continue living in their own homes. Third, we discuss a number of housing options that are currently available to older persons who wish to change their place of residence. Finally, we discuss several current issues relating to the environmental well-being of older persons.

An Ecological Model of Aging

A helpful model for understanding how older persons interact with their physical environments was developed by Lawton and Nahemow (1973). This model, which they call the ecological model of aging, suggests that the same environment may result in very different outcomes for different individuals. Lawton and Nahemow define persons in terms of a set of competencies: biological health, sensorimotor functioning, cognitive skill, and ego strength. They note that some older persons are more competent in each of these dimensions than others. One woman of eighty, for example, might be in top physical health, have only minor impairments in vision and hearing, be fully capable of making her own decisions independently, and have a vital sense of inner strength. Another woman of fifty-nine may be suffering from Alzheimer's disease in addition to severe arthritis. She would be clearly less competent than the eighty-year-old in terms of physical health, ability to get around on her own, and ability to engage in independent thinking.

Just as older persons vary in their competencies, so also do living environments vary in how challenging they are. Some environments make great behavioral demands on people, while others do not. Environments that are challenging and make high demands on a person are said to have "strong environmental press." An example of an environment with strong environmental press is an apartment in a warm climate with no air conditioning, steep stairs, an unpredictable water supply, and rodents. An environment with weak press might be a suite in a luxury hotel where all housekeeping, laundry, and meal preparation are done. Little is left for the resident to do but sit back and relax.

Lawton and Nahemow posit that both behavior and affect (feelings and emotions) are a function of the interaction between a person's level of competence and the press of the environment in which he or she lives. When environmental press is average for a person with a given level of competence, the person perceives the environment as neither too challenging nor too weak. In fact, at this point, most features of the environment are hardly noticed at all. The individual engages in adaptive behavior and generally feels good. Persons with higher levels of competence (for example, the eighty-year-old described above) can tolerate higher levels of press than persons with lower levels of competence (for example, the woman suffering from arthritis and Alzheimer's disease). Simply put, those in better health, who have higher degrees of sensorimotor functioning, cognitive skill, and ego strength are better able to cope with more challenging environments than those with lower competence. There is a limit, however, to how much press a person can live with. If competencies remain constant, and the environment becomes progressively more challenging, it becomes increasingly more difficult for a person to maintain positive affect and adaptive behavior. While adaptations can sometimes be made that will make the environment less challenging, some environments are simply too challenging even for the most competent. The result is negative affect and maladaptive behavior.

It is also possible for an environment to present too little environmental press or stimulation, with the result being, again, negative affect and maladaptive behavior. Some highly energetic and competent older persons have retired to planned environments that do not present sufficient challenges and stimulation. The result is often boredom and apathy and a decision that they have not chosen the most appropriate environment for the level at which they function.

An important aspect of the model is that for persons of low competence, environments must be only minimally challenging in order for outcomes to be successful. A wheelchair-bound older person with impaired hearing and poor cognitive skills is likely to fare better in sheltered housing than he would living alone in a large, two-story house. Further, for persons with lower levels of competence, minor changes in the environment are likely to have more profound implications than they will for the more competent. Lawton and Simon (1968) state this principle as the environmental docility hypothesis: the less competent the individual, the greater the impact of environmental factors on that individual.

An older person in robust health with adequate cognitive skills, could, for example, be expected to cope better with a lengthy power failure than a person who was ill and mentally deteriorated. Similarly, a small change for the better (provision of home-delivered meals) could mean the difference between institutionalization and independent living for a woman in poor health, while it would be a minor amenity for someone able to negotiate shopping and meal preparation with ease.

Professionals who work with older persons are concerned with promoting, maintaining, and restoring optimal levels of functioning. This means, in part, that they want those with whom they work to engage in creative behavior while feeling good about themselves and what they do. Thus, looking at an older person's situation from the dual perspectives of his or her strengths and weaknesses and the demands (or press) of the environment can be useful in attempts to help the person modify behavior and/or the characteristics of the environment.

For most people, advancing age does mean decreases in competence as it was defined earlier, particularly after age seventy-five. While declines are often gradual, poorer health and less efficient sensorimotor functioning are common. The Lawton-Nahemow model suggests that individuals experiencing these decremental changes can function best in environments that become less challenging as competence declines. Later in the chapter, we discuss how the homes in which older persons currently live can be modified to make them less challenging. Some older persons, however, find moving a better solution than home modification. Thus, despite the nostalgia attached to her family home and neighborhood, an older woman may be extremely satisfied with a move to a smaller apartment that is easier to maintain as her health declines. At the same time, it is important to remember that radical changes in environment that reduce press to a level that is too low for the individual's competencies are usually ill advised. A healthy, newly retired schoolteacher, for example, who moves to an environment that places low demands on her abilities is likely to become bored and unhappy quickly.

Following the Lawton-Nahemow model, those who assist older persons with their housing needs may perceive their task as twofold. First, they are concerned with helping the older person improve his or her competencies, maintain them, or slow their rate of decline. At the same time, they work with the older person in efforts to decrease (or increase, if appropriate) environmental press to a level that will result in the older person's being able to live satisfactorily and have positive feelings about the environment.

Improving the Fit between the Person and the Environment

It is not unusual for professionals to be consulted about appropriate environments for specific older persons. Sometimes the request for help comes from the older person. Sometimes the request comes from family members, who are afraid for their older relative's safety and well-being if they continue to live where they are. At still other times, the professional is charged with the responsibility of planning a hospital discharge and needs to determine where the older person might best go immediately afterward. Regardless of how the professional becomes involved, the possibility of moving to a new home (at least temporarily) is likely to be raised. Examples of older persons who might be considering relocation are:

- a retired couple in their sixties who find it increasingly difficult to pay steeply rising bills for home heating fuel;
- a recent widow of sixty-four in declining health who finds her family home too difficult to maintain by herself;
- a seventy-five-year-old man, recently confined to a wheelchair, whose current home is not wheelchair accessible;
- a socially isolated but mentally alert seventy-eight-year-old rural woman whom a public health nurse discovers living in a highly unsafe and deteriorated house without central heating or plumbing facilities; and
- an eighty-five-year-old man who has recently suffered a stroke and whom physicians consider too disabled to resume independent living.

An "objective" assessment of the climates, neighborhoods, and dwelling units of all these persons that takes into account their current competencies and resources might well reveal that positive affect and adaptive behavior are unlikely if the people remain in their current residences. Thus, it is extremely tempting for the professional to conclude prematurely that a move is well advised. Such a conclusion is even more attractive when smaller, barrier-free, safer, or supportive housing is readily available. Planning for a move under such circumstances may seem like the logical next step for the older person.

Research evidence concerning older persons and relocation, however, suggests caution, and in some cases, a search for other alternatives. Older persons tend to be emotionally attached to their homes and to express general satisfaction with them, even when they have severely deficient features. The decision to leave a home, even for a new one of objectively higher quality, may well be a painful experience. Change and readaptation are anxiety provoking and stressful at any age. For the older person of limited strength and resiliency, the demands of searching for a new residence, selling a treasured home, packing, giving up possessions that won't fit, moving, and adapting to unfamiliar surroundings and people can be considerably more stressful than remaining in a challenging but familiar environment. It is not unusual for older persons who move voluntarily to suffer from declines in health and morale. Negative consequences of moving have also been found to occur among older persons who were relocated against their wishes because of urban renewal, eviction, rent increases, or involuntary nursing home placement and transfer.

These considerations suggest that the older person's satisfaction with and attachment to his or her current home, the potential stresses of the moving process, a comparison of features of the old and new environment, the competence of the potential mover, and whether the older person views the move as voluntary or involuntary must all be weighed carefully as the professional and the older person consider the advisability of residential relocation. The older person should be actively involved in the decision-making process unless he or she is totally incompetent.

At least one possibility that should be fully explored is whether modification of the home itself or the way the older person lives in it might reduce the environmental press to a manageable level. The retired couple with high heating bills, for example, might find that installing weather stripping, adding insulation, and closing off unused rooms would reduce intolerably high utility bills. The widow whose house is too large for her to handle may be able to receive homemaker services. Alternatively, a home economist or occupational therapist could suggest rearrangement of the woman's living space or different methods of home maintenance that could reduce environmental press.

It is possible that after a wheelchair ramp is installed, the bathroom remodeled, thick carpeting removed, and furniture rearranged, the man confined to a wheelchair may find his home negotiable with relative ease. The stroke victim might avoid institutionalization if he can avail himself of resources such as an adult day-care center, home health care, and support from family members and friends.

One faces a difficult dilemma when confronted with a social isolate, particularly if that person expresses no wish to change her living arrangements. It is unlikely that home modifications can be made that would significantly reduce the physical threats that her current home presents. The professional who considers encouraging a move to improve the woman's safety and physical comfort, however, must bear in mind that the move itself and adaption to new surroundings may have extremely detrimental consequences for the woman's physical and mental health. The risks of a move may, in fact, be greater than those presented by the woman's current environment. One would be well advised to make sure the older woman is well informed about alternative living situations available to her, while refraining from exerting pressure on her to change her living situation.

The modifications of environment and of behavior within the environment just mentioned are but a few examples of how press can be reduced when competence declines. They suggest that careful attention to the specific ways in which the environment presents demands can be helpful in a decision about whether a move or modification is the better choice. Service personnel who are not skilled in comprehensive environmental assessment should attempt to involve those who are, at least on a consulting basis. Bear in mind that community services available to older persons (transportation, homemaker services, home delivered meals, and adult day care) can help reduce press to an acceptable level and postpone or prevent unwanted relocation.

Those who work with the aged should also be aware of other types of programs and services in their communities that assist older persons to remain in their homes. Several of these are aimed at reducing the cost of remaining in one's home when income decreases following retirement. Most states, for example, provide property tax reductions for elderly homeowners. This can be an important resource for low- and middle-income older persons where tax rates are high.

Another option that may allow older persons to stay where they are is home equity conversion. Most older persons are homeowners, and a high proportion of these have fully paid-off mortgages. Their home equity is their most valuable asset, yet they are unable to make use of this asset to meet monthly expenses. In some areas of the country, financial institutions offer loan or sale plans that enable the homeowner to make use of his or her equity while remaining in the home. Under loan plans, the bank or savings and loan association sends the homeowner a monthly check, using the home as collateral against the loan. The financial institution is repaid, with interest, when the house is sold after the older person's death. In sale plans, the financial institution actually buys the older person's property, and rents it back to the older person for life. Few older persons have participated in home equity conversion programs thus far. Legal arrangements are complicated, and many older persons are reluctant to become involved in a program that is still being tested and refined. Others view their home as the primary inheritance they will leave to their children, and do not want to diminish its value. Although still experimental, home equity conversion may become a well-accepted way for older persons to stay in their homes while boosting their retirement income.

For some older persons, the cost of home energy makes remaining in their homes prohibitive, particularly in the winter months. Low-income elders can benefit from government-sponsored low-income energy assistance programs. The details of these programs vary from state to state, but the intent is to provide the older homeowner or renter with some assistance in paying the costs of home heating and/or cooling. In some areas, privately sponsored programs also assist low-income persons with the costs of home energy.

Another barrier to older persons remaining in their own homes is problems with repairs and maintenance. In a number of communities, home repair and maintenance programs have been developed using volunteers. Assistance with weatherization projects (installing weather stripping and insulation) may also be available.

Housing Alternatives

Contrary to popular opinion, most persons do not change their place of residence in their later years. Older persons are far less likely to move than younger ones. As noted previously, however, professionals who work with the aged are often consulted when older persons are considering alternative housing. The decision to move may be triggered by a number of factors. For some (often recently retired persons in good health with adequate financial resources), change in residence is prompted not so much by the press of their current environment, but by the attractions of an alternative one. Such adventurous older persons may seek the ideal retirement home using climate, opportunities for leisure activities, and proximity to adult children and other relatives as criteria in their choices. For others, relocation is the result of an inability to manage appropriately in an environment that contains too much press for their current level of functioning.

Service personnel who wish to be helpful to older persons considering residential relocations should be aware of the full array of choices available in the communities in which they work. A variety of alternatives is available across the nation, but rarely are all available in a given community and within a price range that a given older person can afford. The following are brief descriptions of the housing choices that may be available to older persons who are considering moving. In this section we discuss two general types of housing arrangements. First, we deal with ordinary housing in regular neighborhoods. Such housing is available to older persons on the same basis as it is to persons in other age groups. Although recreational and other amenities may be available, this type of housing is not designed specifically for older adults and rarely incorporates specific design features and social services intended to create a supportive environment for those in declining health. The majority of older persons live in such housing. A second type of housing, specialized housing for the elderly, is available in many communities. These units have been designed specifically for older persons and tend to restrict their residents to older adults. A variety of special design features and special services are typically available.

"Ordinary" Housing

Purchasing a house or condominium. One option that older homeowners may consider is selling their current house and buying another. Persons who choose this option are often motivated by the thought that a smaller house will require less maintenance and expense than the one in which they have been living. In response to current or anticipated limitations in mobility, they often seek a new house that doesn't require their going up and down stairs and that needs minimal yard work. In a number of cities, condominium communities have been developed that make it possible for residents to enjoy the benefits of home ownership while paying monthly fees for external maintenance and the use of swimming pools, tennis courts, and other leisure facilities. Such communities are often attractive to older persons who wish to enjoy a smaller, more secure home once their children have left home.

Renting an apartment or house. While the vast majority of older persons are homeowners, some 25 percent live in rented units. Typically, persons who rent in their later years are those who rented in their earlier years. However, some older persons who have previously owned their own homes are attracted to rental homes because of the absence of maintenance responsibilities. A number of rental arrangements designed especially for older persons are described below. The majority of older persons who rent, however, live in apartments and homes in "regular" neighborhoods; there are no special features or services designed with their age in mind. Housing counselors suggest that older persons choose rental situations with care, since location, noise level, restrictions on pets and children, and the landlord's commitment to maintain the property can affect how satisfactory the rental arrangement will be.

Renting in transient hotels and boarding homes. Some older persons, particularly single men with low incomes, rent rooms in boarding houses or transient hotels in central city areas. A sizable number of these elderly hotel residents are alcoholics or mentally ill persons and find themselves in these housing situations because there is literally no place else that they can afford. The facilities in which they live are often run down and lack private baths and kitchen facilities. Neighbors may be drug addicts or prostitutes. Although older residents typically qualify for food stamps on the basis of income, they may not be able to take advantage of them because their homes lack appropriate cooking facilities. In cities that are rebuilding their downtown areas, older persons in transient hotels are threatened with homelessness as the hotels and rooming houses are torn down to make way for high-rise office buildings. Social service agencies in some cities are attempting to respond to this problem by purchasing downtown hotels and rooming houses and renovating them to an adequate standard while retaining low rental costs.

Increasing attention is being focused on the homeless and on persons who are only marginally integrated into society. Nevertheless, it remains extremely difficult for low-income older persons without family ties to find adequate housing. Unfortunately, social workers and others attempting to plan discharges from psychiatric and acute care hospitals may discover that low-quality transient hotels or rooming houses are the only alternatives available for the persons with whom they work.

Not all boarding homes and hotels are of low quality. In some cities, under-used hotels have been successfully renovated as attractive homes for older persons who can afford to pay a moderate to high rent.

Some provide meal and housekeeping services and resemble the congregate housing programs described below.

Buying a mobile home. Mobile homes are an increasingly popular housing choice. Older persons considering this choice must give thought both to the type of unit they will purchase and where it will be sited. Some older individuals are interested in the type of mobile home they can tow with them when traveling; others are interested in more permanent siting. Many mobile home communities provide social and recreational facilities, and some (particularly in the warmer states) have been developed to be especially attractive to older adults. In areas where zoning laws permit, older persons often find that living in a mobile home located on their children's property provides for the appropriate combination of privacy and proximity to family.

Living with relatives. A long-standing housing choice for older persons has been to move into the home of relatives. Although some older persons live with siblings or other relatives, they are most likely to live with an adult daughter. Generally, the choice to live with an adult child is not made lightly, and is prompted by the death of a spouse and/ or infirmity. Most older Americans prefer "intimacy at a distance" to sharing a home with the younger generation. Some younger persons put considerable pressure on their parents to move in with them so that they can provide assistance and ensure the older person's safety. When such moves are made against the older person's wishes, problems can be anticipated. As with any move, difficulties with adjustment are likely and these may be compounded if the older person believes he or she is losing independence.

One alternative that is attracting increasing interest in some parts of the nation is called ECHO housing (Elder Cottage Housing Opportunity). Introduced to this country from Australia, where they are called "granny flats," ECHO housing refers to separate, small housing units that can be attached to or placed contiguous to an adult child's home. The idea behind these units is to permit closeness without sacrificing separateness and independence. One form of ECHO housing discussed above is the placement of a mobile home for the older person in the yard of the adult child. Another form involves the use of manufactured housing that can be temporarily attached to a conventional house. The major obstacle to the use of this type of housing is zoning ordinances in single-family neighborhoods. In some areas, activist organizations for the elderly have been successful in changing zoning codes to permit the use of ECHO housing. As our older population grows, this option, which facilitates family involvement with the aged, may find wider acceptance.

Home Sharing Programs

Some older persons find with widowhood and the departure of their children that their homes are too large and too expensive to maintain by themselves. At the same time, they have no wish to move. Other persons, both older and younger, are in need of decent, low- to moderate-cost housing. In response to these needs, agencies in some cities have developed home-matching programs that help persons in both categories find one another and work out satisfactory arrangements. Often house-sharing arrangements involve the exchange of services (housework, driving) for room and board or rent reduction. These arrangements can also result in companionship and a sense of security for the older person. While by no means for everyone, home-matching programs can help both elderly homeowners and other elderly persons in need of satisfactory housing.

Specialized Housing

Retirement villages. In the years since World War II, a number of retirement villages designed specifically for older adults have been developed. Perhaps the best known among these are the Sun City and Leisure World complexes in Arizona and California, respectively. Retirement villages are typically composed of single-family dwelling units available for purchase from a private developer. External maintenance is usually provided for a monthly fee. These villages cater to high- and middle-income older persons in good health who are interested in an age-segregated community that affords many convenient leisure opportunities. Large retirement villages often have swimming pools, golf courses, tennis courts, club houses, and a planned array of leisure activities available for residents. Since they are often located in nonurban areas, they may also have on-site retail shops and services, including banks and hairdressers, for the convenience of residents.

Those who are attracted to and able to afford living in retirement villages are quite satisfied with them. Older persons contemplating moving to a retirement village should consider a number of factors: current and projected costs, location and proximity to family, shopping and services, feelings about living in an age-segregated community, and the appropriateness of the facility if their needs should change. While retirement villages may meet the needs of a healthy, young-old couple very well, they may not be particularly supportive of a surviving spouse in poor health some years from now.

Congregate housing. Often sponsored by religious or fraternal organizations with government assistance, congregate housing for the elderly may provide a number of personal services in addition to an age-segregated living environment. Special design features (wheelchair accessible bathrooms, call bells in units) are usually standard. In some congregate housing units, residents purchase their own apartments and pay monthly fees to cover the costs of services. Others are operated completely on a rental basis. The number of services available varies, but often includes transportation to shopping, light housekeeping, on-site nurses, and planned activities. Some congregate facilities employ social service and recreation staff members to assist residents. It is common for congregate housing complexes to include a common dining area where residents are expected to take at least one meal per day. Congregate housing facilities vary considerably from the luxurious to the more spartan. Generally, however, their purpose is to provide semi-independent living for the aged in a supportive environment. Under Section 8 of the Housing Act, low-income residents of congregate housing may qualify for government rent subsidies.

Life care centers. Life (or continuing) care centers are special cases of congregate housing. They are designed to provide a home for the older person until death, regardless of how ill he or she may become. Typically the person entering a life care center pays a large, non-returnable entrance fee (presumably from the proceeds of the sale of her or his house) as well as a monthly fee. Well residents live in private units, with a wide variety of services available including housekeeping, meals, and transportation. Life care facilities typically include an on-site infirmary for those with acute illnesses as well as a nursing home for those with chronic problems who need full-time nursing care. The idea of moving to a community where one can stay regardless of declining health is appealing to many persons. Unfortunately, developing life care facilities is a risky business, because sponsors are, in effect, gambling on residents' life expectancies. A number of life care projects, even with reputable sponsors, have gone bankrupt, suggesting that older persons considering buying into these arrangements should be very cautious.

Share-a-home. An innovation in housing for the elderly that first appeared in Florida in 1969 and has since spread to other areas of the nation is the share-a-home model. Under share-a-home arrangments, unrelated older individuals who cannot live independently but are not so frail that they need institutional care live together as a family. Typically an outside initiating group, such as a church or social service agency, rents a house that becomes the common residence of the older "family." Monthly payments from family members are used to pay the rent and live-in staff who take care of meal preparation, housekeeping, laundry, residents' transportation, and the maintenance and security of the home. Typically, the initiating group or sponsor provides assistance with financial management, personnel management, and screening of residents. The underlying philosophy for most share-a-home arrangements is to avoid the rigid rules and regimentation of institutions. Rather, the focus is on residents' involvement in self-care, mutual support, and participation in the life of the home.

Foster care. Most state departments of public welfare are authorized to license foster care homes for adults and to place elderly clients in adult foster care. Generally, arrangements are similar to those for child foster care. A family is paid a monthly stipend to provide food, shelter, and other care for an older adult on a temporary basis. Foster care is often the preferred shelter for an older adult who has been the victim of neglect and/or abuse by his or her own family. In practice, adult foster care homes are in far shorter supply than foster care homes for children. Unfortunately, professionals often find it necessary to place older adults in need of protective shelter in nursing homes because suitable foster care homes are not available.

Personal care homes. In some areas personal care (or domiciliary care) homes have been developed for frail elderly persons. Managers of these boarding-type homes agree to provide room, board, and some personal assistance to older persons with a wide range of physical and mental disabilities. While some of these facilities are of high quality, a large number have been found to be abysmally inadequate, taking virtually all of the older resident's pension check and providing poor quality services. Inadequate licensing and regulation in many states contribute to problems. Professionals attempting to find housing for frail, low-income persons should be cautious in making referrals to this type of facility.

Public housing. Beginning in 1956, the federal government has assisted local housing authorities to develop rental apartment units specifically for older persons. In some cases, these are special units for the

g *Older Persons Select Housing*

ntioned earlier, older persons are less likely to move than
persons. Thus, when professionals help older persons with
ental problems, they most often attempt to make the envi-
where the older person already lives more satisfactory.
older person desires to move, however, there are a number of
a professional can be helpful. First, one can help the older
ticulate the characteristics of the new home that he or she
st like to have. Is the older person more interested in special
or the aged or in housing in an ordinary neighborhood? How
s the consumer wish to pay for the rent or mortgage and for
nce and upkeep? How close does the older person want to be
and services? These are but a few of the questions to be an-
a housing search.

a knowledgeable professional can help the older person find
on about a range of alternatives within a community. In a
, there may be many, many choices that meet the older per-
ria. In rural areas and small towns the range of choice may be
row. In any case, human service workers are likely to have
ormation about housing choices, particularly those designed
for older persons. It is generally considered a good idea to
angements for the older person to visit proposed new housing
k with current residents before a decision about a move is
en if the older person is in poor health and is considering en-
acility that provides substantial support, taking the opportu-
sit and choose among several alternatives can ease the stress of
Finally, older persons should have the maximum possible say
cision about where they are going to move if they are at all
f participating in that decision. The needs and wishes of the
son, not his or her family members, should predominate in
about residential relocation.

ould also be noted that not all moves older persons make are
to be permanent. Many older persons enter nursing homes,
ry care homes, and foster homes with the full expectation
will return to their permanent homes after the need for spe-
care is over. This factor should be taken into account in houses and plans should be made for the regular review of the tem-
placement and eventual return of the older person to a
nt living situation.

elderly in housing projects where young
cently constructed facilities tend to rent
housing is a particularly important resou
persons because the government subsidiz
ants are required to pay only a reasonabl
total income for rent, thus making it poss
poverty level incomes to live independentl
lists for public housing units tend to be ve:

The quality of life in public housing v
areas, public housing is crime ridden, an
feel secure. In other areas, public housing i
often consisting of low-rise garden-type
older residents in public housing also vary
Housing and Urban Development views pu
a housing rather than a service program,
available to support the types of services typ
gate housing. Nevertheless, many commun
vative ways to provide services to elderly
Since many housing projects have a large
tached kitchen, these are frequently used as
tion on Aging's congregate nutrition prog
have available to them a hot noon meal and t
interaction with other older persons. It is n
cies eager to reach older clients to send their
ects to provide services. Tenants in public h
better access to low-cost transportation, hom
ational programs, and health promotion prog
private housing.

Institutions. A final category of housing for th
whose primary purpose is to provide physica
vices for older persons who are unable to live
strictive environments. About 5 percent of pers
reside in nursing homes and mental hospitals.
fer to avoid entering institutions if at all possibl
programs developing throughout the nation a
or postponing the need for institutional care.
homes and mental hospitals are important reso
with severe disabilities and for those whose fa
needed round-the-clock care. Institutional care i
chapter 12. We mention institutions at this poir:
spectrum of residential possibilities designed
needs in mind.

Helpi:

As we n
younger
environ
ronmen
When ar
ways th
person a
would n
housing
much d
mainten
to stores
swered

Ofte
informa
large ci
son's cri
quite n
some in
especial
make a
and sp
made.
tering
nity to
movin;
in the
capabl
older
decisio

It
intend
domic
that th
cialize
ing ch
porar
perm

Issues in the Environmental Well-Being of Older Persons

Age-Segregated and Age-Integrated Environments

Special housing options for older persons have expanded in recent years. Entire buildings, complexes, and communities are now available for "mature adults only." A persistent question among gerontologists interested in housing has been whether the trend toward these age-segregated environments, which separate older persons from persons in other age groups, is desirable. One perspective is that residential segregation by age is undesirable. It is said that developing special places for the old to live contributes to negative stereotypes of old age. Older persons who live only near other older persons miss the infusion of new ideas and perspectives that age-integrated living can provide. Younger people, particularly children, miss the opportunities to get to know older persons on a day-to-day basis and to learn from them. Those opposed to age-segregated housing conclude that its end result will be further isolation of the elderly from other members of society.

Others see positive aspects of age-segregated living, particularly for those older persons who choose it voluntarily. Older persons in public housing, for example, tend to feel safer and more secure in complexes composed of their peers. Older persons tend to interact more with neighbors and to be better informed about available services in age-segregated environments than in age-integrated environments. Most older persons who have chosen "older adults only" living situations are satisfied with them, citing reduced interaction with children and young people as an advantage rather than a disadvantage! The services and amenities available at many senior facilities are also cited as advantages of age-segregated environments.

Unfortunately, we just do not have enough information at this point to make a definitive statement about the overall positives and negatives of age-segregated compared with age-integrated housing. Since it is clear that many older persons deliberately seek age-segregated housing and are satisfied with it, we can expect a continuing demand for this type of living environment.

Fear of Crime

A major concern that older persons express regarding where they live is fear of crime. A recent nationwide survey of older persons

(Harris, 1981) revealed that 25 percent of the elderly cite fear of crime as a major personal problem. Many older persons in urban areas feel trapped in the neighborhoods they have lived in all their lives. Over the years, the neighborhoods have deteriorated around them. Those who could afford to move have already done so, leaving behind persons in poor health with limited resources, those most vulnerable to victimization. They live in constant fear in homes that were secure havens in years past. Many exercise extreme caution, installing multiple locks, leaving their homes rarely and then only with considerable trepidation.

Despite older persons' concerns about crime, law enforcement personnel report that older persons are actually less likely to be victims of crime than members of other age groups. They are, however, disproportionately the victims of "larceny with contact," for example, purse snatching. It is important to remember that even minor crimes can have devastating effects on older persons. The young, employed woman who is pushed down and has her purse stolen will likely suffer bruises and inconvenience. The consequences for the low-income eighty-year-old widow who has a similar experience after cashing her Social Security check will probably be considerably more serious. She is more likely to suffer broken bones and be hospitalized, and losing her total income for the month could result in extreme hardship.

There is no easy solution to making living environments safer for older persons. In new construction, designers often use exterior corridors or schemes where only a few families use a single entrance to increase building security. Designs that place entrances and exits in full view of residents, staff, and passersby also discourage unwanted intruders.

Police are usually eager to work with neighborhood residents to develop Neighborhood Watch programs. Crime appears to be minimized in areas where neighbors take an active interest in one another and keep their eyes on the street. Interestingly, a favorite activity of many older persons with limited mobility is watching who enters a building and what is going on in a street. Thus, impaired elders can actually be an important deterrent to criminal behavior.

Police also caution older persons to minimize the effects of possible theft by having their checks deposited directly into checking accounts and keeping only a small amount of cash on their persons or in their homes. Criminals know which days older persons receive Social Security and SSI checks and are especially active on these days. Unfortunately, many of today's older persons have bitter memories of bank failures during the Depression and fear a recurrence more than they fear personal victimization. These elders cash their checks immediately after receiving them and pay their bills personally in cash, making themselves especially attractive targets for street crime.

Neighborhood Characteristics

So far, this chapter has focused on characteristics of individual dwelling units. But, one should also look at the characteristics of the neighborhood in which a home is located in assessing its suitability. Safety is an important consideration. Another is convenience. Since many older persons give up driving and still others (particularly women) have never driven an automobile, neighborhoods and cities planned on the assumption that every adult uses a car are frustrating to the older person who doesn't drive. An ideal situation, one in which an older person can walk or use low-cost convenient public transportation to medical services, the post office, shopping, and the library, is rarely attained in American communities.

The needs of persons who do not drive are rarely adequately considered as cities expand, streets are widened, and the location of services is planned. The professional who works with the aged should be alert to proposed changes in zoning, street location, and traffic patterns that will affect older persons. Advocacy for older persons before a proposed change is implemented can often prevent changing a neighborhood that is a good place for older persons to live to one that is difficult for them to negotiate.

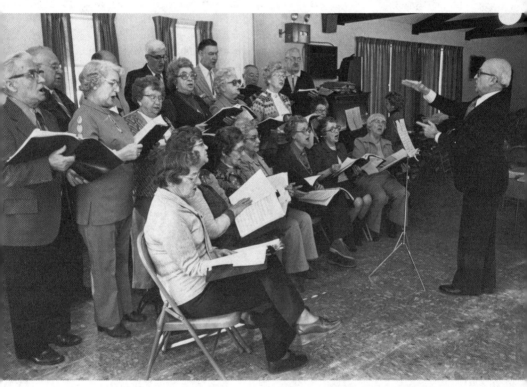

Paul Fortin/Stock, Boston

7

Working with Older Persons

In this chapter, we will present an approach to working with older persons that we think is consistent with our general frame of reference. Our approach owes a great deal to the work of William J. Reid, who writes in the field of social work. We think that his orientation is broad enough to be used by anyone who works directly with older people, regardless of basic professional orientation.

Everybody who works with older people shares an interest in seeing people grow and develop in healthy ways that are personally fulfilling. Social workers are primarily concerned with the *transactions* between individuals and their environments. While other professions and occupational groups have different primary aims, they also have a stake in improving the ability of people to function effectively in their social context—and to act to change the context when a system fails to function appropriately.

The Social System as Organizing Concept

It is convenient to think of human interaction in ecological terms. This implies that the person can be described both as an individual system and as part of other entities that can be said to constitute social systems. Social systems theory has become a popular vehicle for describing people's interrelationships with other important persons and groups in their lives. While the social systems approach is useful, there are some warnings that one must heed in using it. First, there is really no such thing as social systems theory if by that one means a genuine *theory* in the scientific sense of the word. That term *social systems theory* at best denotes a scheme by which one can describe interrelationships. It is not a dependable way of predicting how events will occur. A second problem is that systems are not tightly organized entities. One gets the impression from the term that one is about to hear of an organization as regular as a watch mechanism, but as Gross (1966) has pointed out, systems are rarely very tight, are only partially knowable, and are not fully controllable. Third, there is a tendency for people who write about systems to make them sound as if they are real things when they are simply convenient conceptual ways of describing certain aspects of the way social life works. Given these warnings, social systems theory is still a useful way to talk about people and their interactions because it allows one to describe how people relate to each other and to important social institutions—the family, the economic system, the political system, the educational system, religious and philosophical bodies, and other important social and cultural organizations. Further, it gives one a way to discuss the workings of social institutions and how people either are or are not well served by them.

A social system is composed of people who interact with each other in a number of significant ways. A given human is usually involved in a number of social systems. Anderson and Carter (1974:7–28) have identified four basic functions of social systems: the exchange of information, the exchange of meaningful relationships, the exchange of emotional energy, and the exchange of goods and services. Some systems are characterized as open because they are seen as growing and changing. Closed systems are those that are not receptive to new elements; they are seen as relatively static. Most social systems are said to be organized with some kind of authority structure that resembles a hierarchy. The system literature does not ordinarily describe social systems as having democratic authority structures, but there is no reason why they cannot be so described.

Two terms frequently used in connection with system organization are *entropy* and *synergy*. Entropy is based on the second law of thermodynamics. It says, basically, that closed systems tend to run out of energy over time because they do not receive new energy from outside the system. Open systems are often said to be synergystic, that is, they grow in energy because of new inputs from time to time.

Most systems are said to be goal directed. These goals can be either manifest (out in the open) or latent (unstated and concealed). Within most systems, the parts are specialized in function. A useful analogy (but one not without limitations) is the multipurpose medical clinic. Some of the physicians, nurses, and technicians specialize in the prevention, diagnosis, and treatment of disorders of the eye, others in the gastrointestinal system. Still other specialized teams may be interested in the mental and emotional life of people. While each unit may have a specialized purpose, ideally the whole clinic is interested in the health of the patient and each contributes a particular expertise to the patient's well-being. Of course, there is an implicit assumption that if one sees well, has a good digestive system, is psychologically healthy, and so on, the whole patient is well served. On the other hand, we all know from experience that specialization in a clinic sometimes means that concerns for the whole may be overlooked because concern for the patient becomes fragmented and no one is keeping track of the overall goal. This kind of fragmentation does occur in other social systems as well, and human service professionals need to be vigilant in their efforts to reduce these occurrences.

A good bit of a system's time is spent in what is called boundary maintenance. This means working out the rules and procedures and keeping the system functioning within them. This process occurs on both a formal and informal level. A system tries to reach what is called a steady state. This is not necessarily a static condition, since there are always things that cause the system to change and adjust. The basic idea is that a functioning system should be able to deal with the shocks and changes inherent in human existence and to maintain a balance in an uncertain and shifting world. Communication is said to be a basic process in a social system. Communication is a way of exchanging information, symbols, goods, and services. Systems are said to occasionally interface with each other, meaning that they get "hooked up" for the purpose of making an exchange. Feedback is an important communications process. Contrary to popular usage, feedback does not mean a simple reply to another's statement or question. It refers to a process that moves back and forth between systems. It may help to use the analogy of a boxing match, with each fighter punching and counterpunching in response to the other. Socialization is also an important process in social systems. It is the way in which one is taught the "rules of the game" and becomes used to them.

While this is not a full explanation of the complexities of the application of social systems theory to human affairs, it is sufficient for our purposes.

Our basic stance in working with older persons involves thinking of human beings (and the social entities with which they interact, e.g., family, friendship groups, and social institutions) as open systems—continually growing and changing over time, interacting with other social systems by making various exchanges with them. Too often, older people are tacitly assumed to be closed systems, gradually wearing down over time. While this may be physically true, it is not an accurate way to conceptualize the total functioning of the older person. A few severely disabled older persons may indeed be describable as closed systems. In general, we think it is better to begin work with older persons on the assumption that they can be seen, potentially at least, as open systems.

Recognizing the Strength and Wholeness of the Older Person

In earlier chapters, we have emphasized the notion that older persons are survivors, and that in surviving, older persons have had to develop some real strengths on which we can draw. We want to reiterate this view here, because it is something that in practice is often overlooked. Since we think that much of what can be done to assist older people depends on one's attitude toward aging, we believe an essential part of evaluating the situation of a given older person is to look for strengths. Since we are using the systems analogy, this means that one ought to look primarily at how the older person *functions* rather than confine the evaluation to static characteristics. One of us was once given some advice about buying used cars. The advice was to forget how many miles were on the odometer (which may have been changed anyway) and to concentrate on how well the car actually worked. It is this emphasis that we wish to communicate here. Many older people may have become wrinkled and worn by life. They may even have missing parts! The question is, given all that has happened to them, how well do they run?

There are many older people who have learned to cope with poor health and deficiencies in financial status, social position, and environmental supports. Despite these difficulties, they go on. The importance of this kind of durability should not be underestimated.

It is not uncommon for those who work with people to be overcome by their own values when they look at the life situation of those with whom they have a service relationship. One example from our experience involves a public health nurse who routinely reported parents for child neglect when she found the house less clean than a surgical suite. Despite the best efforts of a number of people, it was impossible to enable this particular nurse to see that a spotless house was not the most important factor in providing a home for children. In fact, it may not be an important factor at all. It can even be argued that neatness can be harmful if the parents are so rigid about neatness that the family cannot use the home for normal activities.

In order to describe the notion of looking at strength, let us take you on a visit to the home of Henry and Deborah Gilmore. We do not claim that they are typical, but only illustrative of the points we want to make.

The Gilmores live in an older house in one of the older parts of a medium-sized city that might be in New York, Georgia, Iowa, Missouri, Colorado, Oregon, or elsewhere. Henry Gilmore is seventy-two, a retired factory worker. He has arthritis, and there are days when it is difficult for him to get around. However, he manages. He tends an extensive garden, which provides the Gilmores with much of their food. Occasionally Mr. Gilmore sells some of the surplus for pocket money. Mostly, he gives the excess produce away to friends and neighbors. Mrs. Gilmore (not Ms. in this case—see the discussion in chapter 2) worked for years as a salesclerk in a discount store. She is vague in discussing her age, but she is clearly of the same generation as her husband. Her heart isn't what it used to be, and she is on daily medication that includes a diuretic, which helps eliminate the excess fluid in her system, and one of the digitalis-like drugs that stimulates her heart. Like many older people, the Gilmores have learned to share the household chores, and they manage fairly well. Together, the Gilmores receive about $900 a month in Social Security benefits (Old Age, Survivors, and Disability Insurance), and they are, of course, covered by Medicare. In addition, both receive small pensions that total around $300 a month, and they have a small savings account of around $10,000.

The Gilmores have two children. The elder, a daughter, is a secretary for an insurance firm in Cleveland and is married to a high school social studies teacher. The daughter and her family visit once or twice a year, and she writes home fairly often and telephones about once a month. The younger child, a son, is a mail carrier and lives in town. He is married too, and he and his wife get together once or twice a month with the older Gilmores and are available for assistance when needed.

The Gilmores keep pretty busy. When the garden doesn't need attention the grass needs cutting. Since the home is old it always needs repair, and the Gilmores' limited income often means that repairs are delayed—unless they are major—so the house goes a little too long between paint jobs, there's always a leaky faucet somewhere, and the furniture has seen much better days. At least, the house is paid for, and the taxes are low.

The Gilmores attend a Methodist church, but they do not take as active a part as they used to. They go to an occasional movie, but most of the movies they see are a bit of a disappointment (except for those made by Steven Spielberg, which remind them of the way movies used to be), so they don't make the effort they once did. They occasionally play euchre (a card game that was popular in their youth) with another couple very much like them and whom they have known all their lives. They watch television in the evenings, but usually go to bed early. They do a little fishing when the weather is nice, but don't care whether they catch anything. They used to take their son's children with them to community events, but the grandchildren are pretty well grown now and have their own interests.

Are there services that you think the Gilmores should have? We'll come back to this question later, but first we want to try to give you some perspective in which to view this situation.

As we suggested earlier, the crucial question is not how old the Gilmores are or how they look from your personal perspective, but how well they function in *their* context. We would view the Gilmores' functioning as an open system that is still growing and changing. This does not mean that the Gilmores live a perfect life. One's eye is immediately drawn to several things. First, the Gilmores' house needs repairs. Their income, while above the poverty line, is not enough to allow them to buzz down to Cancun for the winter holidays. Their health could be better, and they certainly do not have the kind of social life that most younger persons would desire. Taken by themselves, these things might be seen as signs of entropy—of slowing down and increasing isolation from new inputs.

We are not worried by the Gilmores' situation. There are strengths that far outweigh the difficulties. The Gilmores are survivors. They manage in their own way and do not exhibit any great areas of discontent. The house, though old, and the furniture, though worn, are theirs. They have enough income to support their lifestyle and have obviously never been part of the jet set anyway. They have learned to share the necessary housekeeping chores (a good idea for couples of any age) and although some things are let go, they are not major problems. The Gilmores maintain contact with other systems—the family, some old but good friends, and their church. While there are some activities they no longer do to the same extent that they used to, they have things to do that permit them as much activity as they want.

In short, while we might not wish to live our lives as the Gilmores do, there is no good reason for intervening in their life unless they request services. Their family system is intact and functioning, and they interact with other systems in entirely appropriate ways. This does not mean that the Gilmores and those like them will not need or request some services in the future. It does mean that we should not urge services on them when they are not needed. An agency that works with older people may want to inform the Gilmores about the services that are available, should the need arise, but the agency should not aggressively force services on those who do not perceive the need for them.

We do not believe in a planning or service approach that does not consider the wants of the clientele as a primary factor. If older citizens complain that their services are inadequate, it is a different matter. It is clear to us, however, that services imposed because of another's vision of what *ought* to to be are questionable. We would prefer to work with people on the assumption that they should actively participate in matters that affect them, unless they are demonstrably incompetent or destructive to others or themselves. In plain words, if people are satisfied and it does not hurt anybody for them to do what they are doing, we should let them alone!

Much has been said about prevention in recent years. Why not think about the Gilmores, and others like them, in a preventive way? Would it not make sense to begin intervention *before* they exhibit difficulties? At first glance, this seems like a very good idea. There are certainly a number of things one can do to prevent future difficulties. As we have said earlier, one can prevent some health problems through exercise, good diet, the avoidance of cigarette smoking, and the following of other health and safety rules. Certainly people ought to have a will, some insurance against catastrophes, and a good umbrella! As a society, we should do all we can to provide information and education that will enable people to protect themselves from problems, and to know enough about available services to apply for them when they are needed. However, it is possible to go too far with preventive services in a politically free society. A few years ago, one of the authors heard a speech by a mental health professional who proposed that it be mandatory for all primary schoolchildren to be screened for mental health problems. If the screening found situations that *might* lead to mental health problems in the future, he argued, treatment (by law, if necessary) could begin immediately, thus preventing serious mental illness.

There are three serious problems in this kind of thinking. First, except in gross and obvious ways, we do not know enough about the development of mental and personal disorders to prevent them. Clearly, it is bad for people to have inadequate diets, poor medical care, bad housing, and abusive relationships. It is good social policy to have services available that are responsive to consumer wants. However, prevention of specific problems on an individual level is difficult. In the case of the Gilmores, who can tell what intervention would be most preventive? Second, even if we knew how to prevent future difficulties, there is not enough money or personnel to do everything that might be done. In a world with unlimited funds and an absolute commitment to caring for human needs, one could, of course, provide a lot of services. However, we do not live in such a world, nor are we likely to do so anytime soon. Therefore, it is necessary to set priorities in order to make the best use of the resources that *are* available. In practice, this means that agencies and institutions tend to make their services known and then respond to service requests, rather than forcing services on people. This is not necessarily a bad way to organize and deliver services, since consumer demand avoids the third problem with prevention—paternalism.

There is something inherently undemocratic and Big Brotherish about forcing services when they are not requested. Consider your own reaction to people who, over the years, have decided that they know what is best for you! Even if they turn out to be right, one resents the intrusion to some degree. Some human service providers have "helped" people whether they wanted it or not. As often as not, this has been based on notions of the public interest or the common good that do not come from the consumer. The trouble is that no one actually knows what is in the public interest. Or, rather, there are conflicting views on the nature of the common good. Our bias is that the safest course to take is that consumer demand is the surest guide to action. We think that agencies should talk seriously with consumers before designing services and offering them to the public. If the consuming public responds favorably, the helper knows that he or she is providing a desired service. If the product does not gain public acceptance, it simply may not be needed.

We believe that older people (or younger people, for that matter) should have maximum control over their lives. This does not mean that older people must actually operate all services pertaining to them, any more than it means that all medical care must be self-administered. It does mean, however, that service delivery should be provided in ways that are responsive to the wants that older people define in their own terms. The danger of paternalism is especially threatening for older people, because many younger people see all older people as childlike and incapable.

Obviously, there are limits to what can be offered, both in cost as well as technical know-how. Within these limits, however, we think that service consumers ought to be treated in the same way a good store treats its valued customers. A good salesperson does not force inappropriate merchandise on a valued customer, but instead, learns the customer's tastes and wants and then responds.

Protective Services

This discussion does not apply to services that are designated as "protective" services, which are provided for by law. Certain agencies are delegated the responsibility for providing interventive services in the case of abuse, neglect, exploitation, or clear incompetence. It is true that protective services are paternalistic to an extent, but they are deliberately so. Protective services represent a sensible trade-off of individual freedom for social protection. Because abuse and neglect are defined in law, the agencies that offer protective services are subject to public scrutiny and review and thus are accountable via the political process. Further, protective services require the application of due process of law, and consequently, both victim and perpetrator have legal protection. We see this as an entirely different matter than bureaucratic paternalism, which is harder for the public to affect directly.

Clearly, the Gilmores do not need protective services. They are mentally competent, and they are not abused or exploited. An outreach person could offer them services, or a health and welfare agency might advertise available services in the customary way, but there is no need to eagerly press services on the Gilmores. If the community wants to expand an existing service or offer a new one, it should be done after carefully assessing the people who will want to use it. A well-designed needs survey can save an agency a lot of time and money and can help aim the available service resources in genuinely needed directions.

The Other Side of the Coin: Mrs. Nelson

The Gilmores are getting along well enough for us to end our visit with them. However, there are older people who do not have comfortable situations. Mrs. Nelson is one of them. Although she is not an actual person, her situation is real in principle.

We have made the point that most older people generally have reasonably good health. Mrs. Nelson, however, has had a stroke. She was found by her mail carrier lying on the front porch of her house. The mail carrier dialed 911, got an ambulance, and also managed to reach Mrs. Nelson's daughter, who is a police officer. Mrs. Nelson has been divorced for many years, and her ex-husband lives in Seattle. He remarried years ago, but keeps up with the daughter he shares with Mrs. Nelson. Mrs. Nelson is seventy-five. Her daughter, Eileen, is fifty and lives in her own apartment on the other side of town. Eileen is now a lieutenant in the police force and works an extraordinarily demanding schedule. She is single. Mrs. Nelson had a brother, but he has been dead for five years. Other than a stray cousin or two, all of whom live in distant cities, no other family exists. Mrs. Nelson has only recently moved here from Seattle in order to be near her daughter. She has not really had time to become acquainted. Consequently, she does not have the kind of friendship system that many older people have, so it will not be possible for her to count on the help of her neighbors.

Fortunately, the stroke was a mild cerebrovascular accident (CVA) and not a severe cerebral hemhorrage, so Mrs. Nelson has a good prognosis for recovery. However, she may have some residual effects for a while. In the short run, Mrs. Nelson may well need some help.

First, her family system, while intact, is a small one. Her ex-husband is no longer anything but a peripheral part of it. He lives a good distance away, and has established a new family. He may have some small residual affection for Mrs. Nelson, as divorced people often do, but it is not much beyond a few memories of the good times. One could not, and should not, expect any help from him.

Mrs. Nelson's daughter is supportive of her mother. However, she has a demanding job and keeps irregular hours. Many working women are caught in this kind of a bind. Therefore, we have two problems immediately. Because of her stroke, Mrs. Nelson, seen as a personal system, is partially dysfunctional, and she does not have the practical support of a large family system.

Before we go any further with Mrs. Nelson's situation, we want to discuss some principles of helping that we will use in discussing her case example as well as the others that we will talk about in the next three chapters.

Principles in Serving Older Persons

Reid has described the theory behind the service process in some detail (Reid, 1978). We will abstract some principles from his work in order to complete the general orientation that we will use in subsequent examples. We will also add our own view of the service process, which we believe is consistent with Reid's approach.

We have already described and used a simple systems approach in looking at the situations of the Gilmores and Mrs. Nelson. Systems thinking focuses on human beings as functioning entities that grow, develop, and change or, alternatively, stagnate. The systems approach offers us a perspective by which we can visualize human beings as dynamic entities that interact with other entities in the process of getting on with the business of living.

The Purpose

The phrase, "getting on with the business of living," which we use often, is intended to denote the idea that living is a purposeful activity. In promoting a positive view of aging, we are particularly interested in helping people cope with the tasks that life presents. While this is not the place to go into a long philosophical discussion, we have some existential leanings. Consequently, we do not think that life has predetermined ends—other than death, of course—so we generally believe that each person must work out his or her own sense of meaning. The implication is that a common human need is to acquire a sense of mastery, competence, and effectiveness in life. Our job is to help people cope with life and survive as long as they can as well as possible while observing the rights of others to do the same. We think that nearly everyone who helps people can agree with this view, even though they may not have arrived at it from the same starting point.

Of course, there are limits to mastery of one's life situation. People are not gods. They are finite and limited in their powers and in their ultimate achievement. But within those limits, people have the potential for growth and development as long as they live. We believe that it is our task to do what we can to provide opportunities for growth, development, and mastery for all of us, because we share a common human condition. We also believe that we are all accountable to our fellow human beings for our actions, and this provides a moral obligation to be concerned about each other.

The Helping Relationship

While there is a general obligation that we owe each other as fellow creatures, there are special helping roles that people assume in complex societies.

All of us have had some experience in helping someone. Most of the time, our experiences have involved friends or family. Working with people in a service organization is quite different. We help our friends and our families because we have an ongoing emotional relationship with them. They often help us too because that is the interactional nature of friendship and good family relations. We have a long-term commitment to these reciprocal relationships, and we have a large personal stake in them. In a human service context, we do not have the same kind of ongoing, personal relationship that we have with our friends and relatives. The relationship is a more generalized one, and there is considerably less passion in it.

Professional roles differ from those of volunteers. The professional makes his or her living from the work; the volunteer does not. The professional brings years of training to the task, while the volunteer generally learns his or her role in a quasi-apprentice situation. The professional generally is able to perform a range of different functions while the volunteer usually has a specific responsibility.

This is not to argue that the professional is morally superior to the volunteer. The persons who are volunteers in one organizational framework may be professionals in another. In the context in which they are the professionals, they will undoubtedly carry more responsibility than in their volunteer roles. We all have different talents, and we often use them in more than one way in the human community.

The Deliberate Helper

Whether professional or volunteer, certain principles apply. First of all, it is necessary to have a clear view of what one is trying to do. We have consistently taken the position that one ought to have in mind the interests of the person being served. There is a service orientation in which the professional is educated. The volunteer must learn to approximate this orientation through on-the-job training and experience. Both the volunteer and the professional must operate in a deliberate and purposive way that is focused on service acts. Neither should expect the kind of emotional reciprocity with the consumer that one has with friends and family. In human service occupations, the satisfaction comes from doing the job well, not from an intimate, personal relationship. Persons who are engaged in human service occupations must be able to do what they do in a consciously deliberate manner. They must be aware that the consumer will not always like everything that happens in the helping process. Years ago, one of the authors watched a physical therapist who was encouraging an older man to walk after he had a stroke. The patient complained of the pain and annoyance. If the physical therapist had not had a professional attitude, she might have allowed the patient to avoid the pain. However, she knew that if the man didn't exercise, he would probably lose some muscle function. She asked him if he wanted to walk again. He, of course, said he did. She explained to him that it was essential that he start moving as soon as possible, and that it would hurt at first, but that as he got stronger, the pain would lessen. The patient thought a minute, then returned to the parallel bars. He groaned with pain throughout the therapy session, but the therapist kept encouraging him, and he finally finished the exercise. She did not allow the patient's immediate pain to interfere with her professional duty, nor did she become immobilized by the patient's discomfort. She remained brisk, efficient, and supportive the whole time. You should also note that the therapist carefully asked the patient if he wanted to walk; she did not force the exercise on him without his consent.

It would be a mistake to think of the professional attitude as cold and unfeeling. One must have personal warmth in order to render useful human services. At the same time, one must learn to deliver fairly impersonal service. Impersonal is not intended to mean "mechanical" or "disinterested." It does mean that the person being served should receive good service that is directed toward a goal that the consumer considers desirable. Along the way, the consumer may have to suffer some pain, and the professional must accept that without being unduly bothered. Professional service also means that the likes and dislikes of the person offering the service are irrelevant. We cannot offer services only to people we like or who are like us. Our job is to provide services for those who want them without needing to receive emotional gain from the person being helped.

Of course, there are occasions when one's likes or dislikes are so strong that they interfere with providing service. When that happens, one's supervisor will probably recommend finding a way to cope with these feelings or ask that someone else provide the service. If an individual's likes and dislikes are based on feelings of group superiority of a racist, sexist, cultural, or other negative bias, he or she should avoid service occupations and volunteer experiences until he or she has gained a more accepting attitude toward the variations in the human condition.

Essential Characteristics of the Helping Process

Compton and Galaway have surveyed the literature on the helping relationship and concluded that there is a common set of characteristics inherent in deliberate helping behavior (Compton and Galaway, 1984:219–51). Essentially, one must be able to have a positive regard for people. This involves the ability to accept the fact that human beings are not perfect. Others may not make the decisions that we would make under the same circumstances.

The helper should be able to regard the legitimate wants of those he or she would help as important goals. The helper should also be empathic. In Compton and Galaway's words, this means that the helper should be able to "enter into the feelings and experiences of another—knowing what the other feels and experiences—without losing oneself in the process" (Compton and Galaway, 1984:236). It is deadly to say to another, "I understand how you feel"; the idea is to *show* understanding, not to verbalize it. We can never be certain that we know exactly how another feels, but we can demonstrate that we have understood what the client has communicated by sensitive and thoughtful behavior.

Persons who are building a service relationship with others also need to communicate warmth and a nonjudgmental attitude. This does not mean that a helper has to approve of everything the person being helped has done. It does mean that one must respond to the strengths and positive aspects of the person, and not make global moral judgments about the totality of the individual. It is possible, with education and experience, to learn a fundamental respect for human beings without approving of acts of cruelty, meanness, and exploitation.

One other essential quality (often called congruence in the literature) is a consistency of behavior toward the person to be helped, that is, a kind of steady and dependable presence toward the client. Service providers should not blow hot and cold from one day to the next, but must learn to give a consistent performance, much as an actor in a long-running play must do; the consumer should be able to count on the helper's consistency.

Helping persons also must learn how to handle their authority and power. Ordinarily, we do not think of people in human service fields as having much authority or influence. However, human service personnel do have areas of expertise and they also have access to resources. The important thing is that these things are supposed to be used to benefit the client, not to enlarge the ego of the service provider.

The Client or Patient as Valued Customer

We compared the proper attitude of the helping person to the way in which a good salesperson approaches a valued customer. While we have had some colleagues react negatively to the analogy between customer service and the role of the helping person, we still think that it is a good one and that it is consistent with Reid's approach. We suspect that the trouble is our critics do not understand how a good salesperson functions.

In a first-class store, a successful salesperson learns to know the customers. Knowing a customer includes knowing enough about him or her so that the salesperson can given competent service. A good clerk does not "dump" inappropriate merchandise on a valued customer, but genuinely tries to help the customer make selections that will be consistent with the customer's lifestyle and personality. A good clerk will tell valued customers when a sale is coming, particularly if the customer has wanted an item if the price came down. A good clerk will also tell a customer when new merchandise is coming. He or she will even refer a customer to a competitor if the competitor has a good buy on something the customer wants. A good salesperson will not encourage a valued customer to select merchandise that is too expensive for the customer's budget or too extreme for the customer's taste. In short, a good salesperson tries to know what the customer wants and tries to help the customer get it at a good price. A good salesperson learns to offer a service to a customer that enhances the customer's ability to function more effectively in his or her social milieu. This is basically what anyone in human service does. Of course, the motivation is different. The good clerk wants to ensure repeat business, while the human service worker wants to enable people to live a full life, so the analogy is not perfect. Our point is that the human service worker can take lessons from the good clerk about being consumer oriented. In order to reinforce this point, we will often refer to "service consumers" instead of the more familiar "client" or "patient." We want to emphasize the idea that services ought to be consumer oriented. Let us translate our view of helping people as customer service into a simplified version of what has become known as the task-centered approach.

People come to a service agency, clinic, hospital, or other health and welfare facility because there is something they want and don't have. People come together in groups for the same reason. A community hires planners, managers, and service delivery people with the same end in view: the community wants something it does not now have. While motivation is a complex question, it can be seen in these simple terms for our present purpose.

Helping persons are there to aid others in achieving legitimate aims within the limits of their resources and abilities. The first thing to do is to sit down with the consumer and agree on the specific want. Generally, a person's wants have some relation to reality. While we have known individuals whose wants were totally unrealistic, most people want something that is perfectly legitimate. Their expectations of the amount of time and effort involved in meeting their wants may, however, be unrealistic. If the consumer wants something that is completely unrealistic, we cannot be of much help. Helping persons soon learn to tell realistic wants from wholly inappropriate ones, although we admit that there are times when this is difficult.

At any rate, we must first determine the specific want of the consumer. We then have to consider what we can do to assist the person in achieving his or her goal. There are limits to what we can do, and these must be honestly shared. A major factor limiting what can be done lies in the purpose and function of the agency or institution in which the helper is employed. Assuming that the consumer has come to the right place, the helping process can go on. If the consumer has come to the wrong place, it is important that the helping person refer the consumer to the right place rather than just send him or her out the door. Far too often, we have seen clients or patients "cooled out" of what was supposed to be a helping system, and given no direction about where to go with their problems. We do not consider this good practice.

If the service consumer has come to the right place, the second task is to explore the alternatives available. These may involve some kind of service directed at the wants of the individual, or they may involve efforts directed toward some other person or institution.

Simultaneously, we must size up the consumer. What are his or her strengths? What is he or she able to contribute to the achievement of the goal? What can we do within the limits of our abilities and resources?

Next, the service consumer and the helper must agree on a course of action. This involves selecting from among the alternatives available and agreeing about what will be done and by whom. This agreement constitutes a kind of contract that both parties are pledged to honor, pending necessary revisions.

Both the helper and the service consumer, then, should carry out the terms of the contract and work toward accomplishing the goal that has been mutually agreed upon. If all goes well, the task is accomplished in a reasonably acceptable time, and the activity with the consumer can be terminated. Naturally, we hope that the consumer's wants have been satisfied, so it is hoped that both consumer and service provider will agree that the service was worthwhile. After all, we want the consumer to come back if further service is needed or if another problem occurs.

While the discussion above was directed toward helping the individual, the same principles apply if one is offering service to families, groups, or a community.

We take quite seriously the principles that underlie this version of the task-centered approach. We think we have put a greater accent on the role of the consumer than most human service professionals. Take, for example, the matter of evaluation. In most descriptions of service evaluation, the person who delivers the service decides whether progress has been made. In our view, this decision should rest heavily on the judgment of the consumer. While we will not debate this issue here, we will point out that it is technically possible to design consumer-oriented service evaluation. We think it is imperative that this be done.

In summary, we suggest that service providers focus on what Reid calls acknowledged problems. These are problems that the client or patient (or family, group, or community) has explicitly stated and for which he or she wants help. To attempt to provide help with a problem that the client does not acknowledge would be, in Reid's view, a violation of the client's rights. The client or patient usually wants help with specific problems that are related to the specific circumstances in which he or she lives, and there are practical limits to the alternatives available. In the task-centered approach, the person doing the helping talks with the client or patient until the problem is mutually defined, alternative strategies are considered, a decision is made on how to proceed, and both parties agree on who will do what in accomplishing the task.

In this approach, little time is spent in taking an extensive history of the client or patient. The important thing is to define the immediate problem and get to work on it. More traditional approaches to helping operated on the belief that one had to understand the causes of a problem in order to solve it. Reid comments that "It is not necessary to learn why a man is drowning in order to know enough to throw him a rope" (Reid, 1978:42). It is only necessary to establish what lies in the way of solving the problem and to identify incremental steps that can be taken by both the helper and the person to be helped in moving toward a satisfactory solution.

We must caution you that this approach is not as simple as it may sound. We lack the space necessary to discuss all the ramifications of the theory behind these simple-sounding steps, so we recommend that you study Reid's approach if you have not already done so. Our purpose here is to inform you that the task-centered approach is, in our view, the most appropriate one available in working with older people.

The Client as a Consumer

We will take a close look at Mrs. Nelson's situation in the next chapter, but we want to comment briefly on it within the consumer service context that we have outlined above.

As we said, it appears that we will offer services to Mrs. Nelson. The operative word here is *offer.* It would not do to force services on her just as it would not do to try to sell her a garment that she did not want. Whether Mrs. Nelson chooses to use the services available is up to her. The helper's role involves assisting Mrs. Nelson in making her specific wants explicit, helping her examine the alternatives available within a range that is realistic for her, and supporting her as she works out the most satisfactory solution possible given the constraints of her situation.

Even though Mrs. Nelson is improving, she may not be able to resume her old way of life unassisted, at least not right away. Seventy-five is not necessarily too old for a person to resume independent living. We have known people ten to fifteen years older than Mrs. Nelson who are ultimately able to manage quite well. In the short run, however, Mrs. Nelson may need to consider alternatives that might include someone to come into her home to assist or, if that is not possible, somewhere for her to stay until she is better. These alternatives will be explored in more detail in chapter 8.

In any case, it is primarily up to Mrs. Nelson to choose from among available alternatives. One possibility we have not mentioned is that Mrs. Nelson may want to return home immediately upon discharge and may very well refuse all help offered. Unless the case can be made that she is incompetent, it is her right to refuse services.

The helping relationship will not always be a pleasant one. Remember that this is not a social relationship between friends. If it is unrealistic for Mrs. Nelson to return home, we can challenge her view of reality and alert her to the dangers. But then we must stop. She cannot be held in the hospital against her will, nor can the service system force her to accept home services. She could return to her home, be unable to care for herself, and be unable to gain access to any support system. We must recognize that there are limits to what we can do to help Mrs. Nelson and that she has the right to refuse help—even if that refusal results in her untimely death. People who work in the human service system must recognize that clients or patients have the right to fail. Experienced service workers all have had to live with the memory of clients or patients who, despite all efforts, ultimately destroyed themselves in one way or another—by suicide, reckless behavior, or just plain loss of the will or ability to survive. While one is tempted to regard such instances as some kind of personal failure, that is not the case. One cannot be all things to all people, and some situations are beyond human help. Of course, it is possible to save everyone from self-destructive behavior by keeping them locked up or by providing constant supervision, but this is neither practical nor moral. One must be willing to recognize that helping efforts fail and this, like a sale that goes sour, goes with the territory. No helping person wants a negative outcome for a person with whom that person has invested a lot of time and effort, but it happens. One has to accept the fact that there are limits to the effectiveness of even the best effort, and that clients ultimately will and should determine for themselves the outcomes of their lives.

We make an issue of this aspect of the helping process because we have observed a tendency in many helpers to develop what we call the Great Earth-Mother Syndrome. There are those men and women who believe that if they but clasp the "unfortunates" of the earth to their figuratively ample bosoms and do enough for them, all will be well. Helpers with this attitude tend to take over the lives of service consumers and parent them inappropriately.

We think this kind of concern goes well beyond the bounds of good professional service that does not intrude on the rights of the clientele to make major decisions about their lives, even if they are ultimately bad decisions. Service providers cannot and should not live others' lives for them.

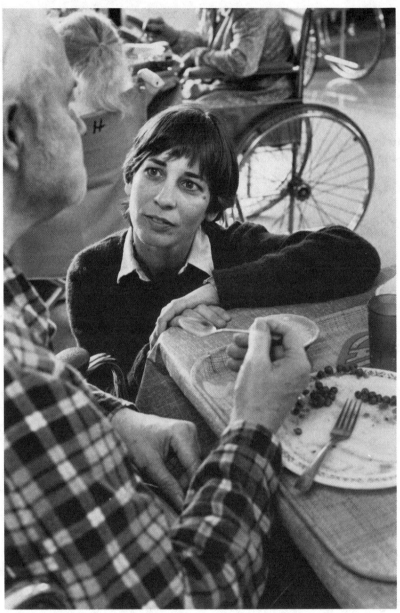

Evan Johnson/Jeroboam

8

Working with an Individual

In this chapter, we will focus on working with older persons when the individual is seen as the primary consumer of services. Subsequent chapters will discuss working with families and groups of older people. Although the principles are similar for all of these potential service consumers, the specific aspects merit special attention.

In a number of circumstances, professionals offer services to older people primarily as individuals; relatively few services are given to the family. We cannot, of course, include all instances in which services are offered to individuals. But here are four examples. First, there are those who have never married and do not have extensive family systems on which they can depend when they need some form of social, emotional, or financial support. Second, there are widows or widowers who have little or no family for various reasons. Third, there are older divorced persons whose position resembles that of the widow or widower. Last, there are older persons whose partners or families do not wish to seek services or are unable to be of help in a given situation.

Implicit in our examples is the assumption that most people turn to their families when they need or want something. In reality, this is what usually happens. The family is a powerful system. Where there is a family and when the family has resources or access to resources, most people turn to it. In many cases, the family is able to provide for its members' wants and needs, or to have some idea about where one can go for specialized services. In many cases, however, the family is small or relatively powerless. Sometimes family members simply do not know what to do or how to do it. In these instances, members needing services must find them as individuals.

We will outline our approach through a series of fictional vignettes. This is, frankly, an old-fashioned approach. Some years ago, the practice of using teaching cases was abandoned in favor of the presentation of theoretical models. The case study approach was discarded because it was believed to be limiting. That is, one might study the case of Mr. Smith, a seventy-two-year-old man with arthritis, in great detail. The trouble was that when we finished training and were prepared to deal with Mr. Smith, he never came in! Instead we got Mrs. Jones, a sixty-five-year-old woman with heart trouble, and we were not prepared for her because she was quite different from Mr. Smith. Because the case approach became so specific, general principles were lost. Therefore, instead of using cases, teachers began to devise theoretical models of the helping process. The idea was that if one understood the theory, he or she could apply it to any specific case. There is a great deal of merit in this approach. The trouble is that most detail is lost. Although students can recite the parts of the model, they often have difficulty making the connections to real people.

By creating fictional cases, we intend to have the best of both worlds. We will present the reader with situations in which we have included enough detail to create the illusion of reality, while preserving the discernibility of our model of providing service (a model is simply a *pattern*) as we go. We will begin with Mrs. Nelson, whom we met in chapter 10. She is recovering from her stroke.

Mrs. Nelson

Although the hospital that Mrs. Nelson is in is small, there is a medical social worker on the staff. Part of the social worker's duties involve engaging with patients in planning for what happens after they are discharged. When Mrs. Nelson had recovered sufficiently to think about leaving the hospital, the social worker stopped by to discuss her future.

When a social worker sees someone for the first time, his or her first task is to build a good working relationship. It is important to remember that this is not a personal relationship in which personal likes and dislikes are important, but a professional one. As we said earlier, the key is to treat the client or patient with the respect and service orientation with which a good clerk in a good store treats a valued customer. The person providing the service must act in a way that encourages a sense of trust and dependability in the service consumer.

In order to build a good service relationship with Mrs. Nelson, the social worker picked a time to talk when the hospital routine was the least hectic. The first conversation might have gone something like this:

The social worker enters the room with a warm but not effusive smile and says, "Good afternoon, Mrs. Nelson, I'm Harvey Smith from the hospital's social service department."

Mrs. Nelson looks up with little enthusiasm, but she does offer her hand to Mr. Smith, who shakes it firmly for a moment.

"Dr. Fitzgerald thinks that you are doing well and that we need to begin to think about your discharge," says Mr. Smith.

Mrs. Nelson nods a little weakly.

"I'll want to go home," she says. The left side of her face is a little slow to move, but her speech is quite clear and her manner is definite.

"Then we'll begin with that as your goal," replies Mr. Smith.

"When will they let me go?" asks Mrs. Nelson.

"Dr. Fitzgerald hasn't committed herself to a definite date yet, Mrs. Nelson. She would like to see you get a little stronger and have some more physical therapy."

"This place must cost the earth. I'm not a rich woman and I can't afford to lie around like this. The money situation worries me," Mrs. Nelson says with more than a hint of anxiety in her voice.

"Don't worry, Mrs. Nelson," says Mr. Smith, with a smile. "I looked at your record. You've got Medicare coverage for both the hospital and the doctor and your daughter told the admissions office that you were covered by a supplemental policy offered by the American Association of Retired Persons. She gave them the necessary information for filing purposes, so you'll be all right."

"Really? Eileen nagged me into buying that policy. I never thought it would do me any good," says Mrs. Nelson with a slight smile.

"You won't have to go to the poorhouse," says Mr. Smith with an answering smile.

"Well, that's one worry off my mind, anyway," sighs Mrs. Nelson.

"Tell you what," says Mr. Smith. "There's just time before your physical therapy to work on one more worry today. Which one do you want to tackle next? Don't make it too big—let's save a big one for tomorrow!"

Mr. Smith has sensed that Mrs. Nelson would respond to this kind of a light touch. Sure enough, there is a slight sparkle in her eyes.

"All right. Tell me your name again, young man, and if I have a complaint, I'll know who to ask for!"

"It's Harvey Smith, Mrs. Nelson. They'll know where to find me."

"All right, Mr. Smith. Now, you said that you had time for one more problem as long as it wasn't too tough. Do you think that you could say something to them about the soup?"

"I can try, but I don't think I'll have much luck. The dietitian has definite ideas about his soup and no one has been able to get through to him yet! Let's try for something easier."

This is enough of this scene to illustrate the points that we want to make, so we'll leave Mrs. Nelson and Mr. Smith now and let them continue their conversation alone.

Things went well in this interview. While interviews do not always progress this well, most of the time they will if human service providers consciously use themselves appropriately.

We began by suggesting an obvious clue to good service. Mr. Smith chose a good time for his first visit. He found a time that was convenient for Mrs. Nelson because he took the trouble to go when she was not scheduled for some hospital routine. Of course, the problem was eased because Mrs. Nelson was in the hospital and the routine was more or less knowable. What if Mrs. Nelson had been living at home? The principle is the same. A good human service provider will try to arrange a time that is convenient for the consumer. This practice ought to be observed by professionals as well as volunteers. Of course, this is difficult when there is the pressure of other clients or patients, but it should be done. Health care providers cannot always schedule carefully, as we all know, because there are emergencies and there are priorities for the use of X-ray machines, CT scanners, and other equipment. This is all the more reason for the human service worker to pay attention to scheduling.

Mr. Smith got the relationship off on the right foot by introducing himself, carefully taking Mrs. Nelson's hand (the pump-handle handshake of the aggressive salesperson is inappropriate here!), and calling her Mrs. Nelson instead of using her first name. He might have asked if she preferred to be called Ms. Nelson, but he took the chance that she was more comfortable with "Mrs." and she didn't correct him. Had she asked to be called by a different name, Mr. Smith would have easily made the transition with good grace.

Mr. Smith stated his business clearly and didn't waste either Mrs. Nelson's time or his own by talking about the weather or the Chicago Cubs' chances for next year. It may suit some people's styles to engage in some small talk when beginning a service relationship, but this is generally a bad idea because it trivializes the purpose of the interview. If either patient or service provider are inclined to chat, this should be done when the main business of the interview is completed.

Mr. Smith did not talk down to Mrs. Nelson as some do when dealing with older people. He shared Dr. Fitzgerald's view of Mrs. Nelson's condition without going into a long, unnecessary discussion. This approach does not usurp the physician's prerogative in any way. Had it been necessary to share any precise information with Mrs. Nelson, Mr. Smith would have told Mrs. Nelson that he would ask Dr. Fitzgerald to stop and talk to her and that he would be glad to be present if Mrs. Nelson wished him to be there.

Mr. Smith was prepared to discuss Mrs. Nelson's major concern. She was worried about the cost of her care. This is not an unusual worry, and patients often need advice. Had the situation been less certain, Mr. Smith would have been honest about her situation. He would have discussed the resources available and offered to explore them on her behalf if she had asked him to do so.

Had Mrs. Nelson revealed a different concern, Mr. Smith would have followed the same general rule of accepting the patient's definition of her major concern.

It is important to note that Mr. Smith did not ask Mrs. Nelson how she was feeling. This phrase has been so overworked that it is devoid of meaning. Medical personnel must ask it, of course, particularly when there is a question of pain, but for other people it is not particularly useful and should be avoided.

As we might expect, Mrs. Nelson wants to go home. Mr. Smith did not raise any question about this, nor should he have. We do not know if it is appropriate for Mrs. Nelson to go home yet, but it is certainly reasonable for Mr. Smith and Mrs. Nelson to start with it as a goal. By accepting Mrs. Nelson's definition of her goal, Mr. Smith has entered into an informal contract to be of assistance in reaching it. Although events may change this contract, it is a good beginning.

Clearly, Mrs. Nelson and Mr. Smith have begun to establish a good working relationship and have even been able to banter with each other by the time the interview is only a few minutes along. Under these circumstances, it is all right to use a more informal touch, just as a good store clerk might do when he or she sees that it will be appreciated. It is clear that Mr. Smith has a serious purpose and that Mrs. Nelson has clearly stated wants that can be discussed and evaluated. Had she been a very hostile, angry person, Mr. Smith would not have treated her lightly, but would have acknowledged her anger and conducted himself differently. It is beyond our present scope to go into all the possible variations that this interview might have taken. It is important to repeat a point, though, before proceeding.

You will recall that in the last chapter, we said that the chief difference between the professionally trained person and the well-intentioned but untrained amateur is that the professional does what he or she does deliberately and in a controlled way. The amateur simply reacts. Sometimes, the amateur reacts with amazing insight. Too often, however, the amateur reacts on a personal basis. When a hostile patient or client is encountered, the amateur tends to react personally without recognizing that the hostility is usually not meant personally. The professional knows that people with problems are often angry, and avoids the unnecessary personal reaction. For this reason, we think that volunteers should receive training in working with people. Although their time is limited and their tasks may be of limited scope, it is important that their services be delivered in as professional a manner as possible. Volunteers should not be simply shoved into a work situation with no preparation or ongoing training.

Mr. Smith has only made a beginning. There is a great deal more to do. Fortunately, the goal is clear, and Mrs. Nelson's wants are not ostensibly extreme. Mr. Smith will encourage Mrs. Nelson to stick with the physical therapy routine. If she regains the necessary functioning to return home and manage by herself, well and good.

But suppose recovery is slow? What alternatives are available? If Mrs. Nelson needs skilled nursing care, she could be referred to a nursing home. Medicare would cover most of the expenses for 180 days, although Mrs. Nelson would be responsible for 20 percent of the cost either from her own resources or from insurance. Legislation passed in 1988 puts a cap of $1,370 on Medicare-covered expenses, so Mrs. Nelson's liability would be limited. A good supplementary policy could cover this amount. Recently, there have been questions raised about the supplemental insurance that is supposedly designed to fill the gaps for Medicare beneficiaries. Some widely advertised policies do not cover nursing home care, so the consumer needs to know what he or she is getting for the money. The safest bet is for the consumer to work with an insurance vendor with whom he or she has had experience and to avoid the more sensationally advertised products.

If Mrs. Nelson does not need skilled nursing home care, she could consider a lower level of care, known as intermediate care, in a nursing home. However, she would have to pay the cost herself, since she is not poor and would not be eligible for Medicaid (which would pay the cost for a low-income person).

Suppose that intermediate care in a nursing home is impractical, or that Mrs. Nelson simply doesn't want to consider it. Many communities now have home health care organizations that qualify for Medicare or Medicaid coverage. As in the case of nursing homes, Medicare's co-insurance feature will require that the consumer be able to pay part of the charge. Again, there is no substitute for good supplementary insurance if one does not have good financial resources.

As a last alternative, Mrs. Nelson may be able to hire the services of a licensed practical nurse who can come in daily. This alternative will not be inexpensive either, but Mrs. Nelson is not destitute, so it is a reasonable possibility, provided that it is not for a long period of time.

If Mrs. Nelson returns to her own home under either of the two conditions above, there are other services that can be of help. We will list and describe a number of them in chapter 11, but we will mention some here. Most communities provide some kind of home delivery service of meals. Meals on Wheels is the best known of these programs, but there are others. In addition, homemaker services are available in most communities. Various personal counseling services are also generally available. In fact, depending on the size and wealth of the community, there may be a number of services that could provide support to Mrs. Nelson if she wants to use them. Some of these services are provided by governmental bodies while others are sponsored by voluntary agencies. Some charge a fee if the individual is able to pay while others are provided at no cost to the user.

We will give the reader a useful hint that we will repeat in chapter 11. Good service providers develop a file of resources in the community in which they work. The major agencies and services are well publicized and easy to know about. However, in every community where the authors have worked, there are local sources for special services. In one community, a local consortium of churches will underwrite the cost of home-delivered meals for people who are not eligible for public assistance. In another, the American Legion Ladies' Auxiliary provides crutches, walkers, canes, or wheelchairs for any community resident who needs one regardless of the patient's financial resources. It is a good idea to keep a list of these services and a current telephone number for the appropriate contact person.

In our list of alternatives, we have not included the possibility of moving in temporarily (or permanently) with Mrs. Nelson's daughter. If both women were to enthusiastically suggest it, it would be a possible alternative. However, since Eileen Nelson has a demanding job with uncertain hours, the social worker and Mrs. Nelson would do well to consider alternatives that would seem less difficult for both Eileen and her mother.

One of the deeply rooted sexist conventions of American society is that the daughter (or daughters) of aged parents is primarily responsible for their care. This responsibility is not conventionally expected of sons, at least not to the same degree. Consequently, many middle-aged women find themselves expected to assume personal responsibility for the care of their parents or other aged relatives. Most daughters will want to be of help, but if they have their own family obligations or are employed, they may be caught between these conflicting responsibilities. If the family has the money, the problem can be handled, of course. However, if a daughter is unable to hire the necessary help, she is often forced to juggle her responsibilities to her own family or career, while squeezing out the time for her aged relatives. This may be praiseworthy from one point of view, but it is a practical nightmare for many. Both the popular press and the professional journals are publishing an increasing number of articles about the burn-out experienced by overburdened daughters. Single women who are employed may especially find themselves singled out for criticism on the grounds that "they do not have families who need them." However, single women may have lives that are as complicated as those of married women, so this criticism is generally unfair.

It is not difficult in this straightforward situation to show the outlines of the task-centered approach. Mrs. Nelson is a competent person who has clearly defined wants that are realistic enough and for whom there are alternatives. Her first task simply involves following a physical rehabilitation routine for which there is a good prognosis. She is well motivated and has enough in the way of resources to manage, although she has no extensive kinship or friendship system upon which she can depend. However, there are social supports available to her when it is time to leave the hospital. The social worker's task is likewise routine, so far. He may need to furnish information about the costs and availability of alternative living arrangements, but this will not be difficult for him. Mrs. Nelson should, on the basis of what has been presented here, be a satisfied customer.

A fair number of helping situations are this simple, and there is no point in making them complicated. There is no need to engage Mrs. Nelson in some form of complicated psychosocial therapy. What she will need is assistance in getting on with the business of living, and efforts that support people in doing that are extremely therapeutic.

However, things are not always this simple, as our next example will show. Mr. MacDonald didn't know what he wanted when he came to a senior citizens' center.

Mr. MacDonald

Mr. MacDonald, a retired automobile mechanic, is seventy-five. He lives alone in a one-room apartment in one of the older parts of the city. He was married twice, but his last wife died five years ago and he has been alone ever since. Mr. MacDonald has three children, two from his first marriage and one from his second. The eldest, Margaret, aged fifty-five, is widowed herself. She works as a checker in a supermarket and shares a small apartment with another older woman with whom she works. The second child, Ralph, aged fifty-three, is a mechanic who works for an automobile dealership in a town forty miles away. The third child, Jeannette, aged forty-five, is married to a salesman. She is a child of Mr. MacDonald's second marriage. She and her husband live in comfortable circumstances in a suburb of Minneapolis, several hundred miles away.

Mr. MacDonald's main source of income is a Social Security check in the amount of $494.50 each month. In addition, Mr. MacDonald earns about $200 a month in interest from a certificate of deposit at a savings and loan. The money represents the proceeds from the sale of the small house in which the couple lived until the wife's death. Under existing rules, Mr. MacDonald is not technically poor. He does not qualify for Supplemental Security Income or food stamps. At the same time, he is hardly among the affluent, and he cannot squander his money.

In a pinch, Ralph can be depended upon to offer limited help to his father. For example, when Mr. MacDonald's toaster stopped working, Ralph bought him a new one. However, Ralph is far from well off, and he is still paying off debts he incurred before his children were raised. On significant holidays, Margaret takes Mr. MacDonald to spend the day with Ralph and his family. Because of the distance involved, Jeannette rarely visits, but she does telephone occasionally. Jeannette was closer to her mother. Since her mother's death, she has not maintained much contact with Mr. MacDonald; she primarily associates with her mother's kin.

Margaret is the child that is emotionally the closest to Mr. MacDonald. Since she lives in the same city, she tries to keep track of him. She stops by to visit at least one night a week and usually she arranges to have a meal with him once a week, either in her apartment or in his.

Mr. MacDonald spends most of his time watching television on an old set that Ralph used to own. Back when he and his late wife lived in a house, Mr. MacDonald puttered around in his garage, fixing lawn mowers for the neighbors and doing the occasional automotive tune-up for friends. Since he has moved into the apartment, he no longer has the space for this, and his tools sit in boxes under his narrow bed. Most of the people that he knew have either died or moved, and Mr. MacDonald has pretty well lost touch with those of his contemporaries who are still in the old neighborhood.

Most recently, Mr. MacDonald has been occasionally dropping into a senior citizens' center that is sponsored by St. Michael's Episcopal church and funded jointly by the church and the United Fund. The center uses space in an old store building next to the church and some of the rooms in the church's parish hall. Mr. MacDonald hasn't stayed long on these visits; he has looked at the newspapers in the lounge briefly and then quietly gone.

Today he will strike up a conversation with one of the volunteers, a young woman who is a premedical student at the local university. Ms. Thompson volunteered because she thought that some volunteer experience would enhance her application to medical school. She has found that the work is interesting for its own sake, and she has become an enthusiastic addition to the regular staff. She is assigned to the entrance lounge because the members and the staff have concluded that it would be helpful to have someone available to greet newcomers and put them at ease.

Mr. MacDonald has just entered the center and is wandering aimlessly around a magazine-covered table in one of the rooms used for general purposes. In one corner, four women are playing bridge. In another, two men are huddled over a table, looking at a set of blueprints for a small boat. Mr. MacDonald is so quiet that the other occupants of the room haven't noticed him, engrossed as they are in their own activities. Ms. Thompson enters the room, carrying a tray with a coffee pot and some cups.

"Good afternoon," she says to Mr. MacDonald. "We haven't met. I'm Beverly Thompson."

"My name's MacDonald," says Mr. MacDonald softly without looking up from the magazines. He seems very shy.

Ms. Thompson takes the tray over to the bridge table and sets it down on a side table. The women nod their thanks, but one holds up her hand for silence, since the play has become crucial.

Ms. Thompson understands the importance of bridge to the four women, who are bridge fanatics, and she quietly moves away and rejoins Mr. MacDonald.

"Would you like some coffee?" she asks. It is part of her job to get a preliminary notion of which of the center's services new people might want to use. In a forward move, this center has opted for this informal type of "intake," rather than a more formal interview.

"No, thanks," says Mr. MacDonald, looking at Ms. Thompson.

"Would you like to sit down and talk to me?" she asks.

"Now what would a pretty young girl like you want to talk to me about?" says Mr. MacDonald.

Ms. Thompson is not offended by Mr. MacDonald's calling attention to her appearance. Although she believes, quite properly, that her good looks are irrelevant, she recognizes that men of Mr. MacDonald's generation were brought up to believe that such compliments are conventionally polite. A younger person without this insight might be offended—or flattered. This is not an important point in itself, but we mention it to emphasize the idea of professional sensitivity and restraint. Had Mr. MacDonald been genuinely offensive, Ms. Thompson would not be obliged to let it pass. It is perfectly proper to take note of overt sexism, racism, or ageism and challenge it calmly but firmly. Such a reaction may not permanently change the thinking of a patient or client, but we do not believe that it is wise to let the consumer think that staff share such biases.

"Come sit and talk to me. I'm sure we can find something to talk about. Tell me about yourself," urges Ms. Thompson.

Few people can resist the opportunity to talk about themselves! Mr. MacDonald follows Ms. Thompson to a corner of the room containing a couple of chairs, a couch, and a coffee table. He gingerly sits on the couch and Ms. Thompson takes one of the chairs. By simply being a good listener, Ms. Thompson gradually draws out of Mr. MacDonald most of the information about his living situation and his family that we have already discussed. He does not talk about his financial situation in detail (people often avoid this) but he reveals enough to show Ms. Thompson that he lives "close to the bone" as our grandparents used to say, but not in dire poverty. Ms. Thompson is struck less by his financial situation than she is by a kind of forlornness she hears in his voice. Her feeling is that Mr. MacDonald's major problem is simply that he is lonely and has little zest for living. However, having had some training for her role, she does not simply jump into action and try to thrust Mr. MacDonald into an activity program. Instead, she decides to ask him what he wants.

At a suitable break in the conversation, she asks gently, "Mr. MacDonald, what might we do for you here?"

"I don't really know," replies Mr. MacDonald.

"Suppose I tell you what we've got. Maybe something will appeal to you," says Ms. Thompson.

"Can't hurt, I guess," replies Mr. MacDonald.

Ms. Thompson begins by explaining that, of course, the drop-in activity room in which they are now sitting is open from 9:00 A.M. to 5:00 P.M. and again from 7:00 to 11:00 P.M. People can come here and write letters (she indicates a desk and chair in another corner), read, play cards, or just chat. There is usually a volunteer who serves coffee, but not always. In addition, a television viewing room is available from 9:00 in the morning until 10:30 in the evening. There is a pool table available during the same hours.

Then, Ms. Thompson lists several groups that she thinks might have an appeal. One involves various arts activities.

"But it's not just busy work," says Ms. Thompson. "These people are quite good and a number of them sell their work at our quarterly exhibits."

"Nope, I'm not an artist," chuckles Mr. MacDonald.

Ms. Thompson isn't discouraged. She describes the group that meets Monday afternoon and studies the stock market. Although they have little money to risk, they maintain a modest investment portfolio. A local bank provides brokerage service at no commission. On Tuesday, there is a preventive health clinic, staffed by family practice residents and senior nursing students from the medical and nursing schools at the local university. On Wednesday, a current events group meets at noon for lunch. Sometimes they have a speaker, but as often as not the participants argue among themselves about the issues of the day. Thursday evening is Five Hundred night (Five Hundred is a card game that is played avidly in this part of the country). A group of aggressive and tireless volunteers have been able, so far, to solicit modest prizes from local merchants. Sometimes, the prizes are odd but usable things that the committee has scrounged from members of St. Michael's and that normally end up in garage sales. On a good night, a winner might go home with a box of laundry detergent and a slightly soiled decorative lamp shade. The lamp shade may show up as a prize again, if it isn't something the winner wants to keep.

On Friday nights, there is square dancing. There are special events, too. Twice a month, a representative from the Social Security office is on hand to answer any questions. At tax time, accounting students from the university are available to help fill out tax forms for those who want assistance.

The center's director, Father John, is the curate (assistant pastor) of St. Michael's. He has a master's degree in social work, and is available to talk to anyone with a personal problem or a problem with any community agency or institution. He also meets with the Member's Council, a body elected by the members for program-planning purposes.

The center is an adult nutrition center, Ms. Thompson explains, and a hot meal is served at noon, five days a week. Instead of charging, the center asks that each participant simply donate whatever he or she wishes before leaving. Sometimes, when the food isn't tasty, the donations are low!

"Well, a nice hot meal wouldn't be bad now and then," says Mr. MacDonald, but he's not enthusiastic. He rises and starts slowly toward the door.

"Tell you what. Why not come for lunch tomorrow? I'll meet you here in the lounge and introduce you to a few people," says Ms. Thompson.

"Well, I dunno. If I don't show up, don't wait for me," says Mr. MacDonald without much emotion.

Ms. Thompson walks with him to the door, still trying to see if there is a clear want that Mr. MacDonald will express. Although she wants to be of help, she recognizes that it would be inappropriate to force services on him. She is quite prepared to see Mr. MacDonald to the door without "making a sale."

"We also are a stop on the Senior Transport Service. If you need transportation to the doctor or want to go to one of the shopping malls, we can provide it."

"You certainly seem to have a lot of things to do," comments Mr. MacDonald politely.

"Our program is planned by our members themselves. Everything we have is in response to members' ideas about what they want. We used to have more transportation services before the bus stopped working," says Ms. Thompson.

"Oh, what bus?" says Mr. MacDonald, stopping and turning to face the young woman.

"It's out in back behind the building. It was donated by the Methodists down the street when they bought a new one, but it hasn't been acting right lately, and we just can't depend on it. Our budget just doesn't stretch for anything major and, frankly, we've just been afraid to ask a mechanic to look at it for fear that fixing it will involve serious money," says Ms. Thompson.

"I'm a mechanic," says Mr. MacDonald in a diffident voice. "At least, I used to be. Would it be all right if I looked at it?"

"Why not? I'll get the keys," says Ms. Thompson, who senses Mr. MacDonald's interest and decides to pursue it.

A few minutes later, the two of them are standing outside the center looking at a vintage bus of the kind that used to be used on short intercity runs.

"It's an old Flxible Flyer," says Mr. MacDonald, his eyes lighting up.

"Wasn't that a sled?" asks Ms. Thompson.

"Naw, that was a Flexible Flyer, with an *e*. See here?" Mr. MacDonald points to the *Flxible* on the nameplate. "These things had Buick-eight engines in them, not diesels."

"Do you think there's anything that can be done?" Ms. Thompson is beginning to have misgivings about straying this far outside the usual duties of her position.

"I worked on them engines for forty years, Miss. I could build one from scratch if I had the parts. Let's see the key!"

Mr. MacDonald climbs into the bus. The interior is in pretty good shape, he notes. Mr. MacDonald sits in the driver's seat and cranks the engine. Amazingly, the engine catches, but clearly not all cylinders are firing. The engine vibrates and shakes and finally coughs and dies. Mr. MacDonald pounds the wheel and laughs out loud.

A young man in a clerical collar comes out of the back door of the church.

"Ms. Thompson? I thought I heard the bus." The young man raises an eyebrow and looks at the young volunteer, but he is smiling.

"Father John, this is Mr. MacDonald. He's a mechanic," explains Ms. Thompson quickly, wondering if she has gone too far out on a limb.

"And a good one, too," says the young man, shaking Mr. MacDonald's hand. "He used to fix my dad's Buicks. Didn't know you lived around here, Mr. Mac."

"Yeah, for about a couple of years since my wife died. So, Johnnie, you grew up to be a priest."

"Afraid so. What are you up to with the bus?"

Ms. Thompson quickly explains the situation to Father John, who nods thoughtfully.

"You really think there's life in the old clunk?" asks Father John.

"Sure is. Blown an exhaust valve and needs a tune-up, but nothing serious beyond that," says Mr. MacDonald.

"How much money are we talking about?" asks Father John.

"Less than a hundred dollars for parts," says Mr. MacDonald. "I know a junkyard that will have the valves, and I can grind the seats myself," Mr. MacDonald says, showing his enthusiasm.

Father John thinks quickly. He can see that he is going to have to square this project with the broker who carries the liability insurance on the center, but he doesn't see any other problems that can't be handled easily. He thinks about who he can tap for the hundred dollars, comes up with three names, and plunges ahead.

"I think I can find the money for the parts all right, but I don't think I can find the money to pay what you're worth," says the priest.

"Oh, that's all right, Johnnie—er, Father John, I can take it out in meals!" says Mr. MacDonald with more enthusiasm than he has felt in years.

"You always called me Johnnie, so there's no reason to stop now, Mr. Mac. There's a vacant room off the back door of the center building if you need a place to put stuff, but what about tools?"

"Tools? Everything I'll need is either home under my bed or I can borrow a few things," Mr. MacDonald replies. "This is an old-fashioned engine, and I don't need the fancy electronic stuff to work on it. Comes to that, I know where I can use some test equipment if we need it!"

"It would sure be a help if we could have our bus back, what with the baseball season coming. We could go to a few games," says Father John wistfully. He misses the trips to the minor league team's games more than the program's participants do.

"I'll start tomorrow morning, if that's all right," says Mr. MacDonald, who seems to have grown taller in the past hour. "And, Miss?"

"Yes, Mr. MacDonald?" says a smiling Ms. Thompson.

"Mebbe I will see you for lunch tomorrow."

It took three weeks, but the bus was running smoothly by the time the minor league season opened. The bus might have been fixed earlier, but as Mr. MacDonald worked on it, other members found out about it and became involved in the project, slowing it down a bit. Mr. MacDonald accepted the "assistance" with good grace, surprisingly, but the bus project was delayed on the days when some brought their cars by and asked the old mechanic to listen to them. The back room of the center now has a couple of homemade tool benches in it, a small lathe, and a drill press. And almost every afternoon, several older men and women can be found with their heads bent over a carburetor or an alternator.

Discussion

In this vignette, we deliberately "salted" some principles that we want to discuss. First, we intentionally created a senior citizens' center that may sound a bit out of the ordinary. In a good bit of popular literature, we are exposed to a stereotypical activity center where the participants are engaged in things that have been planned for them by a well-meaning but paternalistic staff. Notice that, since we have created this one according to our own preferences, the activities have been planned by the members themselves. There is no "artsy-craftsy" busy work, nor is there the ubiquitous kazoo band. There are no terribly expensive programs either, because the center simply does not have unlimited funds. However, it has been possible to meet at least some of the members' wants.

We have devised a novel form of "intake" for our center. Of course, while at some point it may make sense to do some recording of information for various purposes, it is not necessary to take a history and formally admit newcomers to the status of case. We think it makes sense to provide a painless entry into the center's program, and to have a drop-in situation that allows people to move at their own pace.

Of course, Ms. Thompson is a "good clerk." She treated Mr. MacDonald as if he were a valued customer. She spent some time getting to know him in an informal way. She quite properly told him about the center's programs as a good clerk might display the store's merchandise. But mentioning the bus was pure luck. We included the story about the bus in order to make two more points.

First, one of the things that the center did not have was a program that offered the members an opportunity to be of service to someone else. We hope that the Members' Council will take this up at their next meeting! Many older people have accumulated knowledge, wisdom, and skill. A good senior center should provide opportunities for them to use what they know or can do, either as volunteers or on a paid basis. Some centers maintain a job-locating service or provide volunteer opportunities. Not everyone wants to play bridge or argue politics. Some older people are happiest getting their hands dirty. One of the authors has a friend who is in his late seventies. This man has enough money for his material needs, but he also wants to be useful. He does a lot of freelance work making window displays for a local upscale clothing store and gets paid for it. He also volunteers a great deal of time to his church. He can paint, lay tile, and do sophisticated carpentry. He is happiest when he is physically active. Recently he said, "I hope the day will never come when I can't work at something." Fortunately, there is work to be done.

The second point we want to make is that our mythical center has a director who is flexible and willing to try things that are out of the ordinary. Far too often, we have experienced the cautious administrator who has no imagination and who is uncomfortable trusting the judgment of the consumer. In the hands of such a person, the program becomes inflexible, hidebound, unresponsive, and dull.

In this example, Mr. MacDonald was treated as a human being. A want was identified, even if it was by accident. He wanted to do something useful. This was possible in this case, although it would have been more complicated had he not been well known to Father John.

While there was no "talk therapy" in the usual sense, we believe that this is a therapeutic situation in which important psychosocial service was successfully rendered.

Mrs. Brown

Mrs. Brown is what is popularly described as a bag lady. She lives on the streets most of the time, but sleeps at the Salvation Army shelter on stormy nights. She carries virtually everything she owns in shopping bags, piled into a shopping cart that she has "liberated" from a supermarket parking lot. Her age is indeterminate, but she is clearly not a young woman. She has been brought to the mental health clinic for evaluation because of a court order. The police picked her up wandering in the middle of an open-air restaurant, annoying the customers during the lunch hour. She claimed that she was looking for her hat. When the officers tried to remove her from the restaurant, she fought with them and created quite a scene. When brought before the court, her public defender and the assistant district attorney worked out a plea bargain that would send her to county jail for thirty days on the disturbing the peace charge, while the assault on a police officer charge would be dropped. The judge, however, was concerned about Mrs. Brown's mental condition, so he requested a mental health evaluation for her before he actually imposed the sentence. Although she was a familiar local character, she had never created a public scene before. The judge had asked the local mental health clinic to do him a favor and squeeze Mrs. Brown in so he wouldn't have to send her to the state mental hospital, which was 125 miles away. Even so, Mrs. Brown was held for a couple of nights in the city jail before the clinic could work her in.

Paul Boice is a new counselor in the clinic. He was hired primarily to work in an alcohol treatment program, but because of a staff shortage he has been temporarily assigned to interview new patients. He wasn't very happy about this assignment, but he couldn't see an easy way out of it, so he agreed to do it.

Mrs. Brown is escorted into Mr. Boice's office by a matron from the jail. Mrs. Brown sits down and deposits a large, misshapen shopping bag on the floor. The matron leaves the room and goes outside to wait. Mr. Boice looks up.

"Name?" says Mr. Boice, with his pencil poised over a form.

"Ar. Jane Fonda," says Mrs. Brown.

"I understood I was to see a Gladys Brown. Isn't that you?" says Mr. Boice, raising his voice.

"If you knew me name, why did you ask?" snarls Mrs. Brown.

"I just wanted to be sure, Gladys," says Mr. Boice, leaning back in his chair and looking hard at the woman.

"Now, how can we be of help?" Mr. Boice asks pleasantly, with an artificial smile.

"Got a cigarette, dearie?" says Mrs. Brown, looking sideways in what appears to be a caricature of a flirtatious glance.

Mr. Boice has been trying to give up cigarettes, but he has been unsuccessful. He fishes a wrinkled pack out of his shirt pocket and shakes one out for Mrs. Brown. He takes one himself and lights them both.

"How are you feeling, Gladys?" asks Mr. Boice.

"Well, me feet are hurting something wonderful, I've got an arful cough, and I've lost me good hat," replies Mrs. Brown with a serious look on her face.

"We can't do anything about any of that here, Gladys. I mean how are you feeling emotionally?"

"I'm pissed, that's wot. How would you feel if you'd been dragged in here by that storm trooper outside? There I was minding me own business, just trying to find where I'd left me hat and they drag me into

court. Ain't this a free country any more?" Mrs. Brown's tone is thin
and whiny.

"Well, you don't need to use bad language," splutters Mr. Boice.

"Are you a shrink?" asks Mrs. Brown, flirting again.

"I'm one of the counselors here, Gladys. Now if you'll just answer
my questions, we'll get along a lot better. You want me to like you,
don't you?" says Mr. Boice.

"Personally, I don't give a damn whether you like me or not. I
want to get out of here and I want to get on about me business," replies
Mrs. Brown.

"Look, Gladys, I've got to get this information before you can be
diagnosed. Please be more cooperative, or I'll have to get the matron,"
pleads Mr. Boice.

"Oh, all right, duckie, ask your bloody questions!" Mrs. Brown
glares at Mr. Boice, but quiets down.

"How old are you?" asks Mr. Boice.

"I'm over twenty-one," says Mrs. Brown in a coy voice.

"Oh, come on, Gladys, you must be seventy if you're a day," says
Mr. Boice, whose voice has taken on a distinct tremor.

"What to hell difference does it make how old I am, you silly twit!"
shouts Mrs. Brown.

The matron knocks at the door and sticks her head into the room.

"Anything wrong?" she asks.

"No, no, matron. We're just fine, aren't we Gladys?" says Mr. Boice
with a sickly smile.

The matron looks uncertain, but withdraws her head and closes
the door.

We've heard enough to know that things are not fine and that Mr.
Boice is in for a long afternoon. We suspect that if Mr. Boice does not
learn a bit more about his business, he will be in a new line of work
very shortly.

We did not put this incident in this chapter in order to provide a
humorous interlude. Some people with whom one works look and act
in extreme and often ludicrous ways. They are often seen as objects of
humor by the public. One of the authors remembers a woman whose
behavior was quite similar to that exhibited by Mrs. Brown. She en-
dured a great deal of ridicule from children, and most people regarded
her simply as a character. It never occurred to anyone that she was
lonely, frightened, and ill equipped to deal with her environment. We
must often deal with people who are different, even bizarre, particularly in mental health clinics, hospitals, and other voluntary agencies.
Some of these people are old, which seems to make their behavior
more bizarre than if it were seen in a younger person.

It is instructive to look at what Mr. Boice did to get himself into his predicament. This is a protective service situation, and it is not unusual for people who have been brought to a service agency by others to be defensive and hostile. Older people are not an exception, and some of them can be extremely difficult to work with.

Mr. Boice got off on the wrong foot with Mrs. Brown when he failed to treat her as a valued customer. True, she was a vagrant, and an unattractive one at that. But Mr. Boice was in a service occupation. He was pressed into a task that he did not like, but he was an employee of the clinic. The clinic asked him to interview new patients, and he agreed to do it. We are often asked to do things we would rather not do, but there are times when one does his or her best without complaint. This should have been one of those times!

There are several things we have suggested that one who works with older people should avoid. It would have been better if Mr. Boice had stood up and introduced himself when Mrs. Brown came in. It would have been better if he had addressed Mrs. Brown more formally. While we will not discuss the pros and cons of cigarette smoking, we do think that service personnel should avoid allowing patients to "bum" cigarettes, candy, gum, and especially money.

You may recall that Ms. Thompson offered Mr. MacDonald a cup of coffee in our previous example. We think that there is a considerable difference between offering the coffee and allowing a patient to beg things from service personnel. In the case of the coffee, it was part of the agency's strategy to help potential service consumers to feel welcome. Allowing patients to beg things is demeaning to both parties.

Of course, Mr. Boice opened the door for Mrs. Brown's hostile behavior when he asked her how she was feeling. When she became abusive, he reacted in a negative way, something that human service personnel must forgo. Mr. Boice allowed himself to be drawn into a personal exchange with Mrs. Brown and even "lost it" to the extent that he threatened her with the matron. When Mrs. Brown began to use four-letter words, Mr. Boice would have done well to ignore her. Many of the people we are supposed to help will become abusive, particularly if we encourage them by treating them in a less than businesslike fashion. At least Mr. Boice did not reply in kind.

Let us present the situation again the way we think it would have taken place had a more experienced hand been conducting the interview. This time the counselor is Ms. Sharp, who has been doing this sort of thing a bit longer than Mr. Boice.

Again, Mrs. Brown is escorted into the office by the matron. Ms. Sharp is already on her feet.

"Thank you very much, officer. Please sit down, Mrs. Brown. I'm Alice Sharp."

Mrs. Brown sits down and puts her shopping bag near her on the floor. Ms. Sharp sits down too. The matron leaves.

"Mrs. Brown, I know that you didn't ask to come here but, as you know, Judge Parkins has asked our clinic to give you an examination," begins Ms. Sharp in a calm, businesslike way.

"Got a cigarette, dearie?" says Mrs. Brown with a sly look.

"No, I'm sorry, Mrs. Brown," says Ms. Sharp in the same calm, level tone.

"Oh, well, it doesn't hurt to ask," says Mrs. Brown, settling back in her chair.

"Let me tell you what our general procedure is when we do an evaluation, Mrs. Brown," continues Ms. Sharp in the same calm way.

"None of this would have happened if me hat hadn't blown orf. There I was, minding me own business, looking for it in that beanery and they drag me into jail. Ain't this a free country any more?" Mrs. Brown whines.

"I'm sure that it has been an unpleasant experience, Mrs. Brown," says Ms. Sharp.

"How would you feel if you'd been dragged in here by that storm trooper outside?" whines Mrs. Brown.

"You are in a spot, aren't you?" says Ms. Sharp.

"You got that right, dearie! What'll they do to me?"

"I don't know what the judge will decide. I can tell you what we will do, if you are willing for us to do it."

"And if I'm not willing?"

"Then you will be taken back to a holding cell at the jail, and tomorrow morning probably, you'll be taken to county jail to serve your thirty days. The judge held you in city jail so that we could see you for our evaluation. He could have committed you to the state hospital for evaluation, but this seemed the simpler thing to do."

"Can you get me out of this?" says Mrs. Brown with a wink.

"I don't know about that. I'd like to talk to you for a while and get some general information about your situation. After that, if you are still willing, our staff psychiatrist will talk to you, and he may ask you to have some tests," explains Ms. Sharp.

"They gonna stick needles in me?" says Mrs. Brown with an apprehensive look.

"No, the doctor will just talk to you. The tests, if they are used, involve things like looking at pictures and telling a story about them. It may be tiring, but it's not physically painful," explains Ms. Sharp.

"I ain't crazy!" says Mrs. Brown, with dignity.

"I don't think you are either, Mrs. Brown, but something may be wrong, since you did get pretty angry in the restaurant and you did punch out one of the arresting officers. On that basis, we've been asked to take a look at you," says Ms. Sharp.

"I don't really have much choice, do I?"

"I see only two alternatives right now, Mrs. Brown," continues Ms. Sharp. "Either we evaluate your situation to see if we can recommend an alternative to jail, or it's back to the holding cell and your situation will be handled as a straight criminal matter. I'm afraid that's it."

"Suppose I go along with ye. What then?"

"When we have completed our examination, we'll send a report to the judge. To speed things up, I'll give him a short version by tomorrow morning.

"The judge could send you to the state hospital if he thinks you need inpatient treatment. He could release you on probation and order you to come here for treatment. He could simply release you on probation. Or he could just ship you to county jail to serve the balance of your sentence."

"What do you think he'll do?"

"I'm sorry, but I honestly don't know. My guess is that our recommendation will be important, or he wouldn't have bothered to ask for it, but I really don't know. I don't think he'll send you to county jail, but I would guess it depends upon what he thinks after talking to you and reading our report."

"Hell of a thing to do to an old lady," says Mrs. Brown.

"If you had your druthers, what would you like to see happen, Mrs. Brown?" asks Ms. Sharp.

"I'd like to go find me damn hat and go to the Salvation Army and get some supper!" explodes Mrs. Brown.

"I'm sorry that you can't just do that, Mrs. Brown. There are thirty days hanging over your head. What is second best?" asks Ms. Sharp.

"I just don't know," says Mrs. Brown, who is looking really uncomfortable for the first time.

"Are you content with your present life, Mrs. Brown?" asks Ms. Sharp.

"Girlie, I don't have a lot of choices in this life," answers Mrs. Brown, serious now.

"There are alternatives," says Ms. Sharp.

"Sure. The state hospital or some filthy nursing home."

"I was thinking of something else. The Sisters of Martha have taken over the old St. Benedict's Hospital building over on the West

Side. They've converted it into a residence for older people. The rent is low, and they have a cafeteria where the food is inexpensive, but not bad," says Ms. Sharp.

"I told ye I didn't want to go to no nursing home!" says Mrs. Brown.

"St. Benedict's is more than a nursing home. What I'm talking about is a separate wing for people who don't need daily care. You would be free to come and go as you pleased. The sisters will make you feel guilty if you're hard to live with, and they do have some rules. You can't cook in the room, and you have to do your own cleaning. And they will check on you to see that you do, too!" says Ms. Sharp.

"Well, I dunno that I'd like that. Me name was Ryan before it was Brown, and I've seen a lot of nuns in me time."

"I'm not trying to talk you into it, Mrs. Brown. I'm just trying to tell you that there are alternatives. If you want to talk about it later, I'll be here," says Ms. Sharp.

"I'll think about it," says Mrs. Brown, clearly unconvinced.

"Please do. If you want to go over and visit when this business is all over, stop by the clinic and I'll arrange a time when I can go over with you."

"Don't you have to have some clout to get into that place?" asks Mrs. Brown.

"Sure, Mrs. Brown. And I've got some," says Ms. Sharp. "Now how about answering some questions so we can get on with your examination?"

"Might as well, dearie, ask away!" says Mrs. Brown.

Discussion

Of course, since this is our example, we can make it come out the way we want it to. However, we think that most such interviews can follow a pretty similar path, and we have conducted enough of them to be fairly confident about it. Ms. Sharp simply followed what we think to be good practice. She introduced herself, even though Mrs. Brown never called her by name, but persisted in calling her dearie throughout. She knew who Mrs. Brown was, and treated her with dignity from the beginning. She did not become overly familiar, but she was honest and open throughout the interview.

Ms. Sharp did not allow herself to be manipulated, though Mrs. Brown tried several typical gambits to rattle her. You may wonder if it is wise to be so frank about the reason for the interview and the choices that the judge might make. Wouldn't it be better to be more circumspect about the possibilities? Not really. People in Mrs. Brown's situation nearly always know perfectly well what the alternatives are. It is more anxiety producing not to acknowledge them.

Ms. Sharp explained the clinic's role candidly and honestly. There is nothing to be gained by not doing so. She was calm and professional throughout, and did not take any of Mrs. Brown's comments personally. She did, as a good salesperson would, try to find out what the customer might want, and when Mrs. Brown gave an indication that she wasn't sure, Ms. Sharp suggested an alternative to consider. She did not engage in a "hard sell," but she did open the door to further consideration of something that she thought might have consumer appeal.

There's a good chance that Mrs. Brown will be back on the street. In situations like these, judges often suspend the sentence and put the individual on probation. Of course, Ms. Sharp has learned that one can never know what a judge might do, so she is wise in not predicting the outcome. Mrs. Brown doesn't appear to exhibit behavior that the psychiatrist would consider as adequate grounds for involuntary commital. The judge could order her to return to the clinic as an outpatient as a condition of probation. If Mrs. Brown does return to the clinic, she knows that there is someone who will take a professional interest in her. If she is simply released on probation and not required to go to the clinic, she still knows that there is somewhere to go if she is looking for an alternative to her present mode of living.

Summary

In this chapter, we have shown different people working with older individuals in three different settings. In all of them, we have stressed the service orientation inherent in the analogy of the good salesperson. The first rule is to treat the consumer of the service as a good salesperson treats a valued customer, and to do it consistently over time. Those who provide human services (regardless of their professional identification) must treat the people whom they would help with dignity and genuine helpfulness, but they should not become personally involved with them in a way that prevents the rendering of quality service. An essential ingredient in this approach is the acceptance of the client or patient's definition of the problem as the starting point. Sometimes, as we have shown, one must dig around to try to find it, since it may not be clear to the consumer. Sometimes, as was true in Mr. MacDonald's case, one stumbles on the problem by accident. Sometimes one has to fish for it as Ms. Sharp was doing. Usually, the client or patient has a pretty fair idea of what he or she wants to do, as was true of Mrs. Nelson.

The main thing is to work patiently with the service consumer to define the problem and decide who will do what in terms of tasks. Of course, this is not always easy, and often tasks have to be redefined if they cannot be or are not accomplished as originally agreed. The whole purpose is to be of assistance to people who are in the process of getting on with the business of living in ways that seem good to them, and to avoid dominating their lives or patronizing them. Good human service is simple to describe but difficult to do because it demands that we learn to interact deliberately on behalf of others in ways that reduce their dependency and encourage them to consider their options.

9

Working with Families

In chapter 8, we described a number of situations in which older persons were seen primarily as individuals who faced some difficulty in getting on with the business of living. While some reference was made to their families, there was no great importance attached to the family. In some situations, there will be no pressing need to involve the family. In fact, in many cases, there will be no family to involve or, if there is a family, they will not choose to become involved.

As a general rule, however, most older people do have family members with whom they have some degree of contact. In some cases, one who works with older people will find that working with the families takes more effort and time than does working with the older persons themselves.

Older people generally regard their families as support systems. That is, they turn to family members for help of various kinds. Ideally, the family is receptive to the requests of its older members, and it provides moral support, financial assistance, help with tasks, and even personal care when needed. Despite all that has been said about the decline of the importance of the family, for most people the family remains a powerful system for good—or ill—in the lives of most of its members. In this chapter, we will look at the role of the family in a number of situations common in our society. We will also consider how professionals who work with older people can assist the family in supporting its older members.

First we want to make a major point. Please note that we did not say that professionals who work with older people can *use* the family in their work with older people. We have tried hard to promote the notion that the professional should never *use* anyone, but should assist people in continued growth toward their own goals, provided that these goals are realistic and consistent with common decency. Helping people is, whether one recognizes it or not, a moral activity. There have to be some guidelines about what a professional is willing to help another to do. This discussion is especially appropriate when dealing

171

with what one can do to help the family because there are many situations in which the family is struggling with what, at bottom, is a moral issue.

The crux of the issue can be expressed in a question: What do the other members of a family owe to an older person who is unable to be self-supporting, either in financial or social terms? The only answer we can suggest that has any universality is that the other family members should do what they believe they ought to do and what they realistically can do. A corollary is that the family members, once they have committed themselves to be of support, should treat the older person as a fellow human being. The family should accord as much dignity, honor, and personal independence to the older member as they did before he or she encountered difficulties.

Some families will feel obligated to do a great deal for their older members. Others will feel less obligation for various reasons. The professional should not expect families to be able to behave in radically different ways from their previous patterns.

In another era, many states had so-called relative responsibility laws. They are still on the books in some states, but they are rarely enforced. In general, these laws required family members to provide financial support to older members who were in need. These laws had a righteous sound. The problem was that those who were willing and able to support their relatives did so whether there was a law or not. Those who were unwilling to support their relatives could not really be compelled to do so. Although some would like to revive these laws, they have been unpopular, expensive to enforce, and didn't actually bring in much revenue (Schorr, 1980). Further, recent provisions of the Social Security Act (those for Medicaid and Supplemental Security Income) did not require relative responsibility, so most states have given up on the principle.

We have two examples of the futility of these laws. Over forty years ago, one of the authors' parents received a notice from a neighboring state informing them that they were to pay toward the support of an aged relative in that state. At the time, this author's parents were in tight circumstances themselves. They felt guilty because they could not help, but they could not send the money. No attempt was made by the state to collect it beyond the initial notice.

In the second example, an acquaintance of one of the authors received a notice, again from a neighboring state, informing him that he was expected to make a monthly payment toward his mother's Old Age Assistance (this was before 1974 and the change to SSI, of course). The acquaintance was unhappy. He could have afforded to send the money, but since his mother had kicked him out of the house when he was seventeen and told him that she never wanted to see him again, he did not feel obligated to be of help. He was advised to ignore the notice, which he did. No further attempt was made to collect in this case either.

The point is that, as we said earlier, some families want to help their aged relatives and are able to do so. Others are willing but unable, while still others are able but unwilling for a variety of reasons. No amount of legislation has effectively changed this basic situation. The professional who works with families of older persons must accept the family situation for what it is. He or she must not expect radical change in the relationships that have developed over a lifetime.

One other point needs emphasis. Some families want to do too much. This attitude may be motivated by guilt, or it may have to do with the family's perception of what is required by a family in their social position. The motivation is irrelevant, since the effect is much the same. The family that smothers their aged relative, for whatever reason, is difficult. The really poignant cases are those in which the aged relative accepts—or requires—this kind of behavior from other family members. We have not found a consistently dependable method for dealing with these situations. The family, as we remarked before, is a powerful system, and long-term patterns are hard to change unless someone is extremely uncomfortable with the situation.

Family Assessment

When one works with a family on behalf of an older person, the first task is to assess the family strengths and weaknesses as a system. There are a number of sophisticated models that one can use for the purpose. Ours is not very elegant. Because we want to be as practical as possible, we will avoid technical niceties, despite the temptation to construct something more scholarly.

How Does the Family System Work?

First, we must be clear about who we mean when we use the term *family*. Some families are large and include everybody related by birth or marriage. Some sociologists in the 1920s, William F. Ogburn, for example, thought of such extended families as the "normal" family. Later, the concept of the nuclear family emerged prominently in the work of E. W. Burgess, Harvey Locke, and others. The nuclear family consists of two parents and their children. For some family sociologists, the shift from the extended family to the nuclear family as the dominant type in American society signaled a widespread breakdown in the family. For others, Burgess and Locke for example, the shift was only a change, not a disaster. However, it is clear that the notion of the nuclear family as *the* basic family is of limited use. Few families actually involve only the parents and their immediate children. Most families, even though living in different houses and different communities, maintain meaningful exchanges among family members.

Modern family sociologists have added the concepts of the one-parent family and the augmented family to the list of common family types. The one-parent family is the object of a great deal of concern to those in the helping professions. In a way, the term is not as meaningful as it might be, since many one-parent families are really nested within a larger family and interact with it. The term *augmented family* denotes a family type that is less well known. It consists of everybody *considered* to be family even if they are technically unrelated. One of the authors, for example, remembers a woman known as "Aunt" Angie. Supposedly, she was related in some way, but no one seemed to know—or care—what the connection was. She was invited to all family holidays, and could be depended upon for free cookies on the way home from school. Regardless of her formal connection with the family—or lack of it—Aunt Angie was part of the family for all practical purposes.

We do not think that it is productive to worry much about whether the normal family is the extended, the nuclear, or some other form. The plain truth is that we have had—and will continue to have—families of all four patterns among our "customers." While the mix may change, all four are, apparently, permanent family forms—in Western culture at least.

There are other family forms, but we have not included them because their occurrence is relatively rare.

In working with older people, we will take the family as a given on its own terms. As we interact with the family members when service is requested— or required in the case of protective services—we need to worry less about its structure than about its actual function. The situation is the same as the illustration of looking at a used car that we mentioned in an earlier chapter. We should not be too concerned about the form the family takes. The question is, how does it work?

We classify family functioning into two broad categories since we are guided by systems theory. Families either function as open systems or as closed systems. The family that operates as an open system is one in which growth, development, cooperation, and mutual respect are evident. When one works with these families, he or she can sense the vitality that they have.

The family that operates as a closed system is quite another matter. Here we must remind you that *open* and *closed* are not absolute terms, but only approximations. No family is a genuinely closed system, since it may well continue to survive, multiply, and otherwise persist over time. In practice, however, there are families that operate very much in a closed mode. They seem to persist, but not to grow. Their relationships are mechanical and rarely spontaneous. Instead of vitality, these families seem to radiate depression. One gets the feeling that these families are running on past energy, and are slowly running down.

What Is the Older Person's Role?

A crucial factor is the relationship that the older person has with the family. In some families, the older relative has been closely integrated into the family, whatever its form or size. In others, the older person has been on the fringe and is not a vital member of the family group. The relationship of these two dimensions is shown in figure 9.1.

As a rule, we would expect open families to tend to have more highly involved older relatives, while closed families would tend to involve older relatives less. This will not be a perfect relationship, however, since some older people operate on the fringe of otherwise open families while others are highly integrated into closed families.

The utility of this simple scheme lies in assessing the probable direction of the family's efforts when an older person is experiencing difficulties. Open families in which there is high involvement of the older

Figure 9.1

		Type of family	
		open	closed
Involvement of older relative	high	open high	closed high
	low	open low	closed low

members will probably use help most effectively. Closed families in which there is low involvement of the older members will probably require more service and more intensity of service.

What Does the Older Person Want?

We reaffirm our faith in the principle that helping professionals, like good salespersons, are in the business of helping people get what they want, not what we think that they ought to want. When these wants are unrealistic, they cannot be satisfied. Wants, after all, are limited by the possible. Sometimes, people have to adjust their wants to the limits of reality. On the other hand, it is sometimes possible to change the environment enough to make it more supportive of and accommodating to what people want. It is the professional's job to ascertain what the older person and his or her family want, how realistic it is, and what has to be done to move toward the goal.

Some people have a clear idea of a realistic want. Others are unable to define or articulate a want, and the helping professional must spend some time exploring the situation with the older person. Still others want something that cannot be obtained in the world as we know it, and alternatives must be explored.

If the world is not such that people can have what they reasonably want, why not devote serious time to changing the world? People *do* involve themselves in activities designed to change the world—or at least some piece of it; this can be a noble and worthwhile activity. From the standpoint of our concern in this chapter, however, there usually isn't time to change the world in order to better meet the wants of a given person or family. Their pain is immediate, and service must be rendered in the world as it is at the time.

While we would agree that there is a lot of room for improvement, and that we should be involved in social movements that hope to improve the human condition, in dealing with a present situation, we must respond within the limits of reality as they are. Clearly, these limits will affect the achievement of wants.

What causes the older person to move toward a realistic and satisfying goal? This question has to do with strategy. The answer is implied by the preceding discussion. The helping professional, the older person, and the family should, ideally, discuss the problem for which service is requested and examine the alternatives. Ideally, they will all reach agreement on priorities and assignments. That is, under ideal conditions, it works well if there can be agreement on what the older person wants to do, what the family is willing and able to do, and what the professional can do in moving toward a realistic goal. The professional needs to know the relevant medical, social, and psychological data in order to interpret them to the family in a way that enables them to use these data to deal effectively with the problem. Care must be taken in sharing the data, however, to protect the privacy of the older person. Unless the older person is mentally incompetent, his or her permission should be secured before sharing information with any family member. The professional also needs to assess the family's strengths and weaknesses and their ability to cope with the problem.

All of this sounds simple, but the doing takes considerable skill and experience. And, of course, in the real world, we seldom work under ideal conditions. We usually end up approximating this pattern as best we can under the circumstances. Often, the older person's wants may be out of harmony with those of the family. Or the family will want to pursue a course of action that the older person finds extremely unappealing. These complications turn a simple-sounding activity into a complex set of negotiations.

In order to make our points as vividly as possible, we turn to three situations in which the families are involved in events that are crucial to the future of an older member.

The Bensons

The Bensons have come to a family counseling agency on the advice of their family physician. They are concerned about Mr. Benson's mother, who is not present. Earlier in the interview, the family counselor, Paul Bane, gathered the following description of the situation. He had talked to Ralph and Maude Benson, who are in their late forties, their son, Claude, and daughter, Marthe (she calls herself "Marty"). "Mother" Benson, as she is known in the family, is seventy. A year ago, her husband of forty-nine years died of a coronary infarct. Mr. Benson was a hard-driving man who sold insurance. He had not retired, but had continued to operate his independent agency until the day he died. Mr. Benson worked hard, drank more than was good for him, and ate well all of his adult life. Maude Benson has revealed that her father-in-law was also a bit of a rake; she claims that he propositioned her on occasion in his younger days. In short, "Old Mr. Benson" was hardly perceived as a saint—and his character seems to be related to the problem. The younger Bensons think that Mother Benson is not managing well as a widow. She is apparently having trouble sleeping, and she has lost some weight. On occasion, members of the family have seen her crying quietly, but her visits to their house have become infrequent, and she seems to be "drifting away from them" (as Maude Benson puts it). She continues to live in the "big house that old Mr. Benson bought for her" (again Maude Benson's phrase) in one of the more fashionable neighborhoods of the city, but she has not kept up the couple's old associations with friends and organizations.

"Well, that's pretty much the situation," concluded Ralph Benson as he finished the narrative, having had help from each member of the family in the telling.

"So, what do you in the family think about all this?" said Mr. Bane in a warm, even tone.

"Well, it's sure clear that Mother Benson hasn't gotten over Old Clyde's death," said Maude Benson. She was a trendily dressed, attractive woman with what appeared to be a permanent suntan. Her skin had just begun to look leathery. She spent her mornings at the pool and her afternoons and evenings selling real estate.

"We think that Granny's going nuts," said "Marty" Benson.

"Now, Marthe," said her mother (she pronounced her daughter's name "Marta"), "don't talk like that. This is your grandmother we're talking about."

"Well, shit, Mother, it's true." Marthe shrugged her shoulders and tossed her dark hair back from her face with a well-manicured hand. Marthe was a senior in college. She belonged to a "desirable" sorority, and was currently affecting what she believed was a knowing sophistication toward life.

"All right," said Mr. Ralph Benson wearily. In appearance, he was a slightly younger, healthier copy of his father. He had taken over a successful business and, so far, had kept it successful. He did not appear to have indulged himself in his father's excesses. In fact, he showed a great deal of embarrassment when "Old Clyde's" less desirable characteristics were mentioned.

"The point is," said Mr. Benson, turning to Mr. Bane, "We are all worried about Mother Benson and we think that something ought to be done before things get out of hand."

"Has your mother been seen recently by her physician?" asked Mr. Bane.

"Not that I know of. She hasn't told me. I called Dr. Bryant and talked to him, but he wouldn't say anything. His only suggestion was to come here, so here we are."

"I believe that you said that your father has been dead about a year?" asked Mr. Bane.

"That's right," replied Mr. Benson.

"Has there been any other change in your mother's general level of activity?" asked Mr. Bane.

The family members looked at one another.

"Dad, I don't think it's as bad as it appears," said Claude, speaking for the first time. Claude was a quiet, confident looking young man with his mother's lean build, but not her passion for sun worship. Claude had not come into the family business after graduation from college. Instead, to his father's disappointment, he had taken a job with a struggling small firm that produces computer software. Instead of real estate, Claude had chosen to study engineering, and like many of his generation, he was fascinated with computers.

"The truth is, we don't really know how bad it is," said Maude Benson, "since we see very little of Mother Benson lately. She seems to have dropped out of the country club and most of her other social activities since Old Clyde died. It's as if she just isn't part of our life anymore. She rarely comes by the house either."

"What is it that you would like to do?" asked Mr. Bane.

"Well, we wonder if Mother Benson ought to be someplace where she can get help," said Maude Benson.

"Yeah, I told you that Granny was out of it," said Marthe.

"Marthe, dear, we don't like to think of it that way," said her mother with a slight edge in her voice. "After all, we just want what's best for Mother Benson."

"Have you discussed your feelings with Mrs. Benson in any way?" asked Mr. Bane.

"Well, not really," said Mr. Benson. "We didn't want to upset her. We didn't even tell her that we called Dr. Bryant and she doesn't know that we are here, of course."

"Like Dr. Bryant, I'm very reluctant to advise you without talking to your mother and grandmother. Would you be willing to ask her to come in to talk with me?" asked Mr. Bane.

"Well, can't you just tell us what we can do before her condition becomes a public spectacle? After all, we are fairly well known in the community, and we don't want Mother Benson to either go off the deep end or become a notorious recluse," said Mrs. Benson, the impatience showing in her voice.

"No, I really can't," said Mr. Bane gently. "I would not want to advise you on something this important without talking to Mrs. Benson. From your description, she does not appear to be incapable of discussing the situation. I can, perhaps, make it a little easier for you. I can go visit her, if she will permit it.

"Now, I will have to tell Mrs. Benson that you came to me and expressed some concern for her and asked for my advice. I'll need your permission to tell her of your concerns for her well-being. I'll need to ask her about some of the things that bother you, but I'll be discreet, of course. If you are willing for me to proceed on this basis, your task is to tell Mrs. Benson that you have been worried and that you have asked me to see her. If you will do that, I can arrange for a visit. Afterward, I will be glad to sit down with you and see where we can go from there."

"I'll be glad to go talk to Gran, if that's all right," said Claude.

"Well, OK son, I guess it will be all right. You always seem to get along well with Mother, and she thinks a lot of you, I know," said Mr. Benson in a rush. Mr. Bane thought that Mr. Benson sounded relieved.

A few days later, Claude Benson telephoned Mr. Bane with the news that his grandmother would be quite willing to see him any time. Mr. Bane asked Claude to arrange a convenient time with his grandmother and suggested several times that would be best for his schedule. Accordingly, the next morning, Mr. Bane stopped to see Mrs. Benson at her home.

Mrs. Benson met Mr. Bane at the door. She was a slim woman with a clear complexion. Her hair was white and neatly cut in a short, boyish style. She wore a plaid shirtwaist dress that fit her neatly. She greeted Mr. Bane pleasantly and led him into a sun porch off the kitchen.

"I hope that you don't mind talking out here, Mr. Bane. I find this by far the most pleasant room in the house."

"It's a lovely room, Mrs. Benson," said Mr. Bane.

On the coffee table stood a pot of fresh coffee, a plate of croissants, butter, a pot of strawberry jam, and a pitcher of orange juice.

"Please sit down, Mr. Bane, and join me for coffee and a croissant. Have some orange juice. It's fresh squeezed," said Mrs. Benson.

"I'll settle for some coffee, Ma'am," said Mr. Bane.

"Oh, go ahead and put some butter and jam on a croissant, young man. Live a little," said Mrs. Benson with a smile, "I intend to!" She poured coffee for Mr. Bane and herself and put a croissant for each of them on small plates.

"You talked me into it, Mrs. Benson. Thank you very much," said Mr. Bane, laughing.

"I know that this is a business call for you, Mr. Bane, but I don't see any reason why it has to be uncomfortable for either one of us," said Mrs. Benson with a smile.

"You're right, Ma'am," said Mr. Bane, taking his cue from her attitude, and biting into his croissant.

"So my family thinks a few shingles have come off my roof," said Mrs. Benson, smiling again. She put a tiny bit of butter on her croissant and a small amount of jam.

"Oh, it's all right, young man. I know what they think. I'm just surprised that they noticed."

"Ma'am?" asked Mr. Bane.

"Mr. Bane, Claude says that you're all right. And he's the only one of the lot with any sense, so I don't think I need to beat around the bush. The truth is that my poor son, my elegant daughter-in-law, and my misguided granddaughter are boring!"

Mrs. Benson finished the last bite of her croissant, took a sip of coffee, and sat back in her wicker basket chair. She looked at Mr. Bane and smiled.

"I'm not what you were expecting, am I?" she asked.

"Well, frankly, no you're not," said Mr. Bane.

"Claude told me all about your meeting, Mr. Bane. He's a good boy. Ralph looks like his father, but Claude's the one that's really like him. Oh, Claude's not the rakehell his grandfather was, but he's got the drive and the willingness to take risks. I'm glad he didn't go into business with his father. He and his friends may go broke in the computer business—I don't pretend to understand just what they do—but Claude will give it a go. The rest of them are in a rut. It's the curse of the middle class!"

"Mrs. Benson, you're certainly not what I expected. I frankly don't quite know . . ." began Mr. Bane.

"Oh, don't worry about it, Mr. Bane. As I said, Claude reported the whole thing to me.

"First, let me tell you about my husband. When he started in the insurance business, we were in the midst of the Great Depression. You won't remember what it was like, but it was tough. Clyde worked night and day just to keep afloat. Back in those days, he sold a lot of what were called industrial policies. People paid their premiums by the week and Clyde had to go 'round and collect the payments. We lived in an apartment over a drugstore. There was a laundry across the street and they had a flashing neon sign that went on and off all night long. After we made some money and moved out of there, we had trouble sleeping at night because we missed that sign!"

Mr. Bane chuckled with her.

"In those days, few women had real careers. Those that worked had jobs, but not many had what I would call a career. I was an English major in college, and I didn't have a teaching certificate, so I worked with Clyde. I kept our books, did the typing, took the phone calls. He couldn't afford a secretary. Besides, we worked well together. In 1939, when Ralph was born, I quit work. It was, frankly, a mistake. Quitting work, I mean, not having Ralph! I had two more children, you know."

"No, I didn't, Mrs. Benson. I didn't really ask for a family history the other night," said Mr. Bane.

"Yes, I have two daughters. Claire is a doctor—an internist, no less. And Marian is a professor of English at State."

"And you're very proud of them, too."

"Sure am. Of course, I don't get to see much of them, but they write and we talk on the telephone. But I'll see more of them in the future."

"Oh?" asked Mr. Bane.

"Look. Let me tell you a little about my life. That's what you want to know about, isn't it?"

"Well, I should get some kind of a picture of your situation, at least, Mrs. Benson," said Mr. Bane.

"When I quit work, Clyde had to hire a girl to work in his business. He couldn't pay much, so he didn't get much. Things actually got tougher. Then came the war. Clyde didn't get drafted right away, but when he saw it coming, he enlisted in the navy. He was in service for three years. Closed up the office. I had Ralph and Claire to take care of. She was born in 1941. When Clyde enlisted in 1942, I ended up—after he finished his basic training—living in Norfolk. It was no picnic, I'll tell you."

"I'll bet it wasn't," said Mr. Bane.

"After the war, Clyde started over. Marian was born in 1946, and I didn't go back to work. Frankly, Clyde did get a little wild at times, but I really have trouble believing that he made a pass at Maude. She wasn't his type," said Mrs. Benson.

"But you're not saying that your husband was a saint," said Mr. Bane.

"Not a bit of it. He had his faults, all right, but I wouldn't have left him no matter what. My one regret is that I didn't stay with him in the office. I think that, like a lot of middle-class women of my generation, I got boring. Oh, I've no one to blame but myself. I should have hired someone to stay with the kids and stayed right there in the office. I'll bet I could have kept the agency open during the war if I had done that. The women's movement has changed the way we feel about all that sort of thing now, of course. I wish it would have started in 1939!"

"But you do miss your husband," said Mr. Bane gently.

"You're damn right I do, young man," said Mrs. Benson with a slight catch in her voice. "He's been gone a year now, and despite his faults, I loved him. And knowing what I know now, I think I would have been a different woman—and he'd have been a different man. But I wouldn't have wanted him too different. Just a few less drinks and a lot fewer women! But, you see, Clyde, too, hadn't been liberated. He had caught the fever that many men of his generation had. He thought he had to work and drive and push in order to make me happy. He didn't realize that it wasn't the money, it was the work that was fun. And I had gotten out of it."

"You're pretty insightful. Am I wrong to think that, even though you are a very bright woman, you didn't work all this out alone?" asked Mr. Bane.

"You're not unobservant yourself, Mr. Bane," said Mrs. Benson. "You're right. I've been talking to other widows. We think of it as a kind of therapy, even though it's not really a therapy group. We meet at St. Michael's on Tuesday nights. Father John sits in sometimes, but we really don't need him."

"Do you find yourself drifting away from your family?" asked Mr. Bane.

"Not drifting away, Mr. Bane, *moving* away. As much as it grieves me to say it, my son and his family are in a terrible rut. Their lives are so predictable. Ralph goes to work, Maude to the pool, and Marthe—what an unfortunate name—to do whatever she does. The weekends are spent at the country club. Ralph plays golf and Maude plays tennis. Every summer, they will spend two weeks at the beach. In the winter, Ralph and Maude will spend the week after Christmas in Florida. They always stay in the same place. Marthe will snag—and I mean snag—some promising young man who will get sucked into the routine."

"For some people, that would seem to be a pretty comfortable life, Mrs. Benson," said Mr. Bane.

"I know. And Clyde and I started them on it, I suppose, but I don't think that it really was the same for us as it is for them. When Clyde and I made a little money and began to spend it, we looked at it as an adventure. My son's family look upon their life as if it were the only legitimate life that 'their sort' of people should live."

"So what do you want to do, Mrs. Benson?" asked Mr. Bane, again very gently.

"First, I'm going to sell this house, much as I love it. Ralph doesn't want it—well, actually, Maude doesn't want it is the thing."

"Meow," said Mr. Bane quietly with a smile.

"Yes, I suppose it was catty of me, but I am really distressed by how stodgy they have become," said Mrs. Benson.

"So what do you plan to do when you sell the house?" asked Mr. Bane.

"I'm going to look into the advantages of moving to the same town as one or the other of my daughters. I don't want to move in with either of them, but it would be nice to be near one of them as I get older. I'm going to take my time and see which city has the most advantages for me. My daughters are both agreeable, and there's only fifty miles between them anyway, so I'll be able to see more of both of them."

"Sounds all right to me, Mrs. Benson, but I really ought to earn my money for a minute. May I ask you a few questions?" asked Mr. Bane.

"Of course."

"You mentioned that you missed your husband. How has your general health been?" asked Mr. Bane.

"For a long time, I had trouble sleeping and I cried a lot. Dr. Bryant said that it was to be expected."

"Then you have seen your physician?" asked Mr. Bane.

"Not for a while now. I went to him after Clyde died, and he gave me some medication. Mostly, he just let me talk. Sam Bryant has been doctoring the family a long time, and he's not a pill pusher, but a good friend. He suggested the widows' group," said Mrs. Benson.

"Have you lost quite a bit of weight?" asked Mr. Bane.

"How nice of you to notice. But that wasn't grief, young man. That was exercise and diet!" said Mrs. Benson proudly.

"Your family was concerned because they hadn't seen you around as much. Need they be alarmed?" asked Mr. Bane.

"Not for me. I've been busy. I'm studying French and geography— and going to an exercise class!"

"Planning a trip?" asked Mr. Bane.

"Do you have to tell Ralph and Maude?" asked Mrs. Benson.

"No. Before I go, I'd like to discuss with you what I can share with Mr. and Ms. Benson, since I do owe them an appointment. But I'll tell them that they need to ask you about any questions they have."

"Well, if you'll let me have my secret, I'll tell you. In a couple of months, Claire and Marian and I are going to Europe. Claire wants to go to a medical meeting and Marian isn't teaching this summer, so we're going to go and spend three weeks. What's the sense of having money if you don't enjoy it? But I don't want Ralph and Maude to know just yet, because they will fuss themselves unnecessarily about it. They think I'm in my second childhood as it is!"

"And all you're doing is breaking out of a rut?" asked Mr. Bane.

"You've got it, as Claude says!"

"One way to clear the air would be for all of you to sit down and have a good talk with each other," said Mr. Bane.

"I'll do that before I make any serious moves. But frankly, I'd like to get a little further with my plans, if I could. Of course, Ralph and Maude could have kept up with what I was doing if they had really wanted to. Claude knows, but he visits me often."

"And you've sworn him to secrecy, I suppose?"

"Yes. Wicked of me, isn't it?" Mrs. Benson's eyes sparkled and she smiled.

After receiving Mrs. Benson's permission about what needed to be discussed with her family, Mr. Bane left.

In a few days, the Bensons sat down with Mr. Bane again. "Well," began Mr. Benson, "what do you think?"

"Mr. Benson, I don't think that your mother's situation is alarming," said Mr. Bane.

"What?" exclaimed Maude Benson.

"How long has it been since you've talked to her?" asked Mr. Bane.

"Oh, I talk to her on the telephone at least once a week," said Maude Benson.

"How long has it been since you sat down and had a really good talk with her?" asked Mr. Bane.

"Oh, maybe a couple of months, no longer. Ralph, didn't you stop by last week?" asked Ms. Benson, turning to her husband.

"No, I think it was the week before," said Mr. Benson.

"I think you all have lost touch a bit," said Mr. Bane with a smile.

"We know she was feeling badly, but we didn't want to intrude on her," said Ms. Benson.

"It's been hell at the office, and I guess I'd just gotten into the habit of coming home without stopping. I used to stop fairly often right after Dad died," said Mr. Benson. There were signs of guilt in his voice.

"It's the easiest thing in the world, folks; I'm not trying to make you feel bad about it," said Mr. Bane still smiling, "but I am saying that I think that Mrs. Benson seems to be doing well and I don't think that you need be alarmed."

"But her weight loss?" asked Maude Benson.

"Exercise class, Ms. Benson," said Mr. Bane.

"Exercise class! At her age? What can she be thinking?" asked Maude Benson.

"I can't see Granny as a jock," said Marthe with an amused smile.

"I think that your grandmother is a surprising woman," said Mr. Bane, "but I should tell you that she has Dr. Bryant's approval and that Mrs. Benson is exercising well within her physical limits. It's a supervised class for older people at the YWCA."

"At the Y?" asked Maude Benson with just a hint of disapproval in her voice.

"Sure. She's a member," said Mr. Bane.

"Then that's where she's been going?" asked Mr. Benson.

"That's one of the places," replied Mr. Bane.

"Then she's doing some other things, too?" said Maude Benson.

"She's been going to college for the past several months, too."

"Oh, you're not serious," said Marthe. "Why didn't I ever see her?"

"She's been taking some lower division courses. I expect that she was just in a different place," said Mr. Bane.

"But she's got a degree," said Mr. Benson.

"She's just stretching her mind, Mr. Benson. A lot of older people take college courses today," said Mr. Bane.

"But what about her grief?" asked Mr. Benson.

"It appears to be pretty well under control. It's not unusual for people who have lost someone close to them to hang on for a while. I think she's coping pretty well, though," Mr. Bane assured them.

"She really did love the old—Old Clyde, then," said Maude Benson.

"Yes, she did, Ms. Benson," said Mr. Bane, deliberately gentle now.

"I guess we have lost track," said Mr. Benson.

Claude, who had been silent, looked at Mr. Bane and winked. Mr. Bane smiled back.

"What do you think we should do?" asked Mr. Benson.

"I think that you might take your mother to lunch!" suggested Mr. Bane.

"Then she's all right?" asked Maude Benson.

"I think so, Ms. Benson, but she is making a few changes," said Mr. Bane.

"But at her age?" said Ms. Benson.

"Many older people use these years to do things they didn't get around to doing. Your mother-in-law is just doing a bit of growing, that's all," said Mr. Bane.

"Well, I'll be damned," said Mr. Benson, "I guess we'll get used to it."

"I think you'll have to," smiled Mr. Bane. "You might even find yourself growing with her."

The Bensons left Mr. Bane's office partially relieved, at least, but still a bit puzzled. Except for Claude, of course, who was obviously amused. He paused for a word with Mr. Bane after the rest of the family had gone out the door.

"They really don't quite understand, you know," said Claude, "but I'll work on them."

"If I can help . . ." began Mr. Bane.

"You already did. Gran got a kick out of your visit. She really blew your mind, didn't she?"

"She sure did. She's a remarkable woman," said Mr. Bane.

"I wasn't sure what would happen when the family came here. I was worried up to the point where you said you couldn't suggest anything until you talked to Gran. I was afraid they might embarrass themselves by trying to do something uncalled for, and that you might have taken their view of Gran as correct. I knew, though, that if you went and talked to Gran that you'd see that she was all right."

"That's standard procedure. I won't stick my neck out until I see how things are," said Mr. Bane.

They said good night, and Claude left to join his family.

Discussion

This has been a rather long example. Let us examine the principles and issues involved.

First, let us look at the Benson family. They are an upper-middle-class family, and they may be a bit of a stereotype, but they are not terribly different from families that we have known. Few of these families will be seen in community agencies that deal with aging persons or in family counseling agencies for that matter. We have included them, though, for two reasons. First, professionals will see a few families of this type, and this family gives us a chance to remind the reader that not all persons who perceive problems in their relationships are economically disadvantaged. Second, inclusion of the Bensons allows us to raise another question. Should agencies that cater to older people try to restrict (either officially or unofficially) their services to those who are poor or near-poor? We think not. Both tax-funded and voluntary agencies are supported by the public, and the public includes both the poor and the nonpoor. Of course, most voluntary agencies charge fees. Those who can afford to do so should be expected to pay the full rate for their services. Agencies that are supported *by* the public, either through taxes or contributions, should be available *to* the public. Pain is pain.

Ralph and Maude Benson and their daughter approximate a closed system. Clearly, they are in a rut, albeit a comfortable one. Their routine is "right" in their eyes, they lack creativity (on the basis of our knowledge of them, at least), and they have been unable to deal realistically with Mother Benson's desire to chart her own course. The older Mrs. Benson's role has become peripheral to the local family system. Of course, in this situation, Mrs. Benson's lack of participation in the immediate family system is her idea. In other situations, the family pushes older members away when they act in ways that differ from the family's accepted lifestyle. It is not uncommon for older members of the family to become detached as a consequence of widowhood. Both the professional literature and the popular magazines have described the tendency of others, even those in the family, to exclude the widowed from common social interaction.

Mother Benson began to act differently when her husband died. While she displayed some of the symptoms of prolonged grief, it was not as bad as the family thought. Those working with older people often see grief symptoms. Commonly, these include some level of depression with periods of weeping and frequent sighing, loss of sleep, loss of appetite with corresponding weight loss, and sometimes, feelings of unreality. The grieving may also include guilt, the bereaved believing that they failed to do all they should have done for the deceased. Some may be angry at the deceased for dying and leaving them unsupported.

It is hard to draw a line between normal and abnormal grief. DeSpelder and Strickland (1983, pp. 194–195) suggest that grief becomes abnormal when the symptoms interfere with the person's ability to get on with the business of living. Grieving persons normally may be affected by the loss of a person close to them, even long after his or her death. This loss is particularly painful on holidays or important anniversaries.

In the case of the Bensons, the old saying that a little knowledge is a dangerous thing seems to apply. They knew that Mother Benson had lost weight and sleep and that she had fits of crying. However, because they—and she—had put some social distance between them, the family didn't know that the weight loss was not due to grief. Nor did they know that Mother Benson was aware of her grief and was coping with it in constructive ways. It is not uncommon, unfortunately, for family members to develop an unwillingness to talk openly about grief and about their concerns for the grieving. The reader may think it is strange that the Bensons did not simply have it out with Mother Benson and express their concerns directly. In the real world, the reticence to be frank is a common phenomenon. Whether families fear to deal with these matters for psychological reasons or because admitting these problems would constitute a threat to their perceptions of their social status is not clear. The fact is that they often have trouble dealing openly with older family members.

What does Mother Benson want? Note that Mr. Bane asked the family what they wanted, but he did not attempt to satisfy their request until he had talked with the older Mrs. Benson. Note that he carefully spelled out what they were supposed to do to prepare for his visit. Note also that he carefully got both the family's and Mrs. Benson's permission to discuss the situation, and he specified what he would and would not discuss with whom. It is important to point out that professional confidentiality requires that one behave in this way. It is fairly common for older people to find that their rights to confidentiality of information are ignored, that family members often are given information that ordinarily would be considered privileged. If the older person is demonstrably incompetent (and this holds for younger persons too), there is justification for handling information differently, but this clearly was not the case in this situation.

Mr. Bane was careful to determine what Mrs. Benson wanted from life. Although he did not take a formal social history (as many agencies still do), he did encourage Mrs. Benson to talk about herself and to share with him the factors that she considered relevant to her current functioning. Mrs. Benson used the opportunity to engage in reminiscence—a common phenomenon in older people. Elsewhere we have discussed the "life review" and we wanted to include an example of how this might actually occur in a therapeutic relationship. Mrs. Benson, like many real older persons, wants to grow and to live a full life. Of course, she is financially well off and can think in terms of a European trip. In our last chapter, Mr. MacDonald found overhauling an old bus a fulfilling thing to do. A European trip would not have been a likely possibility for him. We cannot deny that a person's socioeconomic status colors his or her wants, and often seriously limits options. However one may feel about this, in providing direct service to an older person, one has to accept it as a fact of life. Service cannot be denied until all the inequalities of life have been redressed, even if one believes that should be done. Besides, who is to say that a trip to Europe is qualitatively better than fixing up an old engine? It depends on how one derives satisfaction from life.

What has to happen in order to accomplish the goals? In this instance, this question is easily answered. Mrs. Benson is a self-starter. But what if we had used an example in which money was tight? The principle is the same. The helping professional and the consumers of service must still determine who will do what and when.

Mr. Bane was professionally courteous to everyone involved. He didn't try to whip the Benson family for their lack of communication with Mrs. Benson. He may have agreed with Mrs. Benson's evaluation of their conventional life, but he didn't say so. Mr. Ralph Benson is not an especially stimulating person. His wife may appear to be a bit of a snob. Marthe is not a highly attractive person. Mr. Bane did not castigate them for their shortcomings. He did recognize that Claude and his grandmother tended to be mutually supportive, and he did encourage them in their relationship.

A good salesperson would have the sense to accept the customers for what they are, and would try to help them buy a satisfactory product. He or she would not expect that current want satisfaction would result in a whole new way of life for them. Nor would a good salesperson expect that the customer should conform to the salesperson's notion of a worthwhile human being. As we saw in the example, the family will probably not be a lot different in the future, but the solution of this problem might make it possible for the Bensons to use help more constructively at another time.

One last point needs discussing. Should Mr. Bane have accepted Mrs. Benson's hospitality, or should he have refused to eat breakfast with her? Earlier we made the point that professionals and trained volunteers should be careful about allowing clients or patients to beg cigarettes, money, and the like because this behavior may be a form of manipulation that the client or patient can use to obtain advantages that are outside the acceptable limits of service. Mr. Bane decided that Mrs. Benson's offer was simply a reflection of courtesy and not an emotional bribe. He was hesitant until this became clear. Many people will offer coffee or some other form of food and drink simply as a matter of courtesy when someone visits their home, even on business. Our rule of thumb is to accept such offers when they are matters of simple courtesy, but to refuse them if they appear to be an attempt to gain emotional advantage. It is our view that alcoholic drinks ought always to be refused, and one is not obliged to accept any food or drink that he or she really shouldn't eat. There are exceptions, and there may be times when it is easier to drink coffee that one doesn't want than to seriously hurt the feelings of an older person who wants to show courtesy.

Let us turn to some other examples of working with older people in which the outcome is less certain.

The Phillips Family

Nedra and Derek Phillips are a middle-aged couple who face a difficult situation. Nedra Phillips' mother, Emily Tyson, age seventy-six, has broken her hip. A heavy woman, Ms. Tyson has responded to treatment moderately well, but it is unlikely that she will be able to manage without considerable assistance. Currently, she is in the hospital, but she is reaching the point where it is likely that she will be seen as having had maximum hospital benefit. Thus, it is time to think about what happens next.

Both Mr. and Mrs. Phillips are employed. Mrs. Phillips, age fifty-four, is a legal secretary. Mr. Phillips, age fifty-six, is a machinist. They are talking with Gertrude Schmidt, the head nurse on the orthopedic unit. Part of Ms. Schmidt's job is to advise families about the aftercare needs of orthopedic patients. Ms. Tyson has been consulted, and has willingly given permission to discuss her care with her daughter and son-in-law. Below is a part of a conversation that Mr. and Mrs. Phillips had with Ms. Schmidt in the latter's office.

"So you see, Mr. and Mrs. Phillips, Ms. Tyson will need some assistance in bathing and getting in and out of bed for a period of weeks. She will also have to have some assistance with exercise in between outpatient physical therapy appointments. Now, I'll show you how you can bathe Ms. Tyson and later one of our physical therapists will go over the exercises with you. I'd like you to spend a few minutes with our dietitian, too, since we'd like to see Ms. Tyson lose some weight," said Ms. Schmidt.

"Wait a minute," said Mr. Phillips. "This is all coming pretty fast."

"I know it's a lot to think about. I'm sorry. I don't mean to rush you," said Ms. Schmidt.

"We want to help Mother. It's just that it's not going to be easy. We both have jobs, you know," said Mrs. Phillips.

"Yes, I had forgotten." Ms. Schmidt paused. "Let's see if we can think this through together."

"A broken hip is pretty serious for someone Mother's age, isn't it?" asked Mrs. Phillips.

"Yes, it is," said Ms. Schmidt gently. "There can be complications all the way from pneumonia to bed sores. Recovery is often slow, and it's especially difficult for heavy people."

"So someone needs to be available to get Mother out of bed from time to time?" asked Mrs. Phillips.

"Yes. She should sit up often in a comfortable chair, and she needs to spend an increasing amount of time out of bed. She can go to the toilet with help, but she won't be able to walk without help for a while, so someone will have to be with her."

"You mentioned exercises. What does that involve?" asked Mr. Phillips.

"There are some exercises that we call range of motion exercises. Someone will have to gradually move Ms. Tyson's legs and bend them for her. She will be given weekly appointments with our physical therapist, but these exercises need to be done every day to help reduce the tendency of the muscles to become flabby and the joints to become stiff," explained Ms. Schmidt.

"And we'd need to do this at home?" asked Mr. Phillips.

"Yes, but the physical therapist will show you how they are done and will give you printed instructions. The instructions have pictures to show how each step is to be performed."

"And she'll need a special diet?" asked Mrs. Phillips.

"Well, ideally, we'd like to see her lose some weight primarily to relieve the strain on her hip and knee joints.'"

"Ms. Schmidt, we really want to help Mother, but I can't quite see my way through this. I don't see how I can handle all this without quitting my job," said Mrs. Phillips. She appeared to be on the verge of tears.

Mr. Phillips reached over and took his wife's hand. The warmth between them was almost palpable, thought Ms. Schmidt.

"There are things that can be done without you quitting your job," said Ms. Schmidt.

"I don't want to see Mama in a nursing home," said Mrs. Phillips in a soft, dejected voice.

"That isn't the only alternative, though," said Ms. Schmidt.

"You know, Miss Schmidt, it's hard for black people to give up on family. At least it's hard for *these* black people," Mr. Phillips said, indicating his wife and himself.

"And I wouldn't ask you to ever do that, Mr. Phillips," said Ms. Schmidt gently. "Let's explore what's available. We need to include Ms. Tyson in the planning, too, but we can take a preliminary look now. I think that it will ease your minds to do that," said Ms. Schmidt.

Ms. Schmidt explained the services available in the community. Mr. and Mrs. Phillips were not poor, and they had been able to save some money in recent years. On the other hand, they were not wealthy either, so there were practical limits to what they could afford. Ms. Tyson's resources included Social Security, which includes Medicare coverage, and a small teacher's pension. The total was less than $500 a month. Ms. Tyson had taught most of her career in small rural schools, and she had never received the kind of salary that would have qualified her for large benefits. Ms. Tyson had been living in a small apartment near the Phillipses' home before she fell and broke her hip. She was still paying rent on it, and, in fact, the Phillipses had been supplementing her Social Security and pension benefits because Ms. Tyson enjoyed having her own place. As they began to discuss the alternatives, the best appeared to be hiring a nursing assistant to supplement the visits from the local home health care agency that would be providing follow-up care. Ms. Schmidt could see that even with both husband and wife working, this wasn't going to be easy.

"Look, folks, we don't have to decide anything today," said Ms. Schmidt, "and anyway, we need to talk it over with Ms. Tyson and see what she would like to do."

A few days later, Ms. Schmidt met with Mr. and Mrs. Phillips and Ms. Tyson on the sunporch at the end of the hall. This gave them all a relaxed place to talk and some privacy.

Ms. Schmidt reviewed with them the doctor's prognosis and the various sets of instructions that the hospital would be sending home with Ms. Tyson. It was expected that Ms. Tyson would be able to walk unassisted in three to four months, but should continue to use a walker until the doctor and physical therapist were certain that she could manage without it.

Ms. Tyson and Mr. and Mrs. Phillips had talked about what Ms. Tyson would do after she left the hospital. Ms. Tyson agreed that it would be nice to stay with her daughter and son-in-law during her recovery period. Mrs. Phillips had engaged a nursing assistant who was willing to take care of Ms. Tyson during the day. The Phillipses believed that they could handle the care at night and on the weekends during the recovery period. They believed that some of their relatives and friends would also be willing to help a bit when things got hectic. There were several members of the family living in town. In the past, the extended family members had been able to count on each other in times of difficulty. Ms. Tyson had suggested that she give up her apartment temporarily and find another one when she was ready to resume independent living.

"I was about to move anyway," she said. "I wanted to find someplace closer to the shopping center since I don't drive. This will give me lots of time to find something I'll like better, and we can use some of my pension money to help pay the nursing assistant instead of paying rent for an empty apartment."

"Now Mother, don't worry about the money," said Mrs. Phillips.

"I'm not worried, Neddie, but you two have done a lot for me already, and I know it won't be easy."

"But you're family, and we don't want you to have to worry," said Mr. Phillips.

"I can see that the family has gotten things in hand," said Ms. Schmidt.

"I think we'll be all right," said Mrs. Phillips. "It's just that people sometimes need a little time to sort things out."

Ms. Schmidt left them chatting on the sun porch.

Discussion

Chronic long-term illnesses often become problems that the whole family faces. Ms. Tyson is fortunate to live in a close relationship with her daughter and her son-in-law. Had the relationship been strained, things would not have worked out this well. This isn't going to be an easy three or four months. Ms. Tyson's care will take a lot of time and it will mean some juggling of the budget. But this is an open, flexible family that is willing to learn and grow. Further, Ms. Tyson is well integrated into the family unit.

Ms. Schmidt recognized the warmth in the family, and she also was able to give the family time to think through their situation. Less sensitive professionals might have pressed for a resolution without waiting for the family to process the situation. As often happens, between appointments the family had discussed the situation and had already taken steps to deal with it.

Mr. and Mrs. Phillips and Ms. Tyson did not want to consider a nursing home. In their view, this would have amounted to "giving up" on Ms. Tyson.

It is true that nursing homes have been used by some families as dumping grounds for their unwanted members. It is also true that some nursing homes are not desirable resources for older people. On the other hand, there are many nursing homes that are well run and can be used as extremely effective resources both for temporary and long-term care. We will discuss the use of nursing homes in chapter 12, and share with you our thoughts and experiences with nursing home selection. Right now it is only necessary to point out that Ms. Schmidt did not press this issue with Mr. and Mrs. Phillips or Ms. Tyson, since they felt strongly about keeping Ms. Tyson's care in the family, and a workable way of caring for Ms. Tyson was possible. Many families feel this way, and it is often difficult to refer families to nursing homes when their use would be appropriate.

If Mr. and Mrs. Phillips are able to manage, this situation will work out. If it does not, the family may have to consider a nursing home until Ms. Tyson is able to manage a bit better. From an outsider's point of view, it might be easier for all concerned and better for Ms. Tyson's physical recovery if she went to a nursing home right after leaving the hospital and moved in with Mr. and Mrs. Phillips when her recovery was farther along. However, the family has worked out its own solution, and helping professionals do not have the moral right to urge a different solution unless the one selected is clearly harmful to the persons involved or the public health. It might have been possible to either intimidate or seduce Mr. and Mrs. Phillips into making a different decision, but it would not have been ethical from our point of view. Since the whole family made a decision, it is best that Ms. Schmidt supported it. If things don't work out, she can help Ms. Tyson and Mr. and Mrs. Phillips to identify an alternative.

This is a family that can be described as an open system. What Ms. Tyson wants is not unrealistic, given the strength of the family. Further, everyone is prepared to do what needs to be done to handle the situation. Unless there are complications, Ms. Tyson should recover and may be able to resume independent living. If she does not do well, Mr. and Mrs. Phillips and Ms. Tyson may need to rethink what they can do, but this situation looks healthy and we would expect a successful resolution.

Mr. Hayes

Mr. Hayes is eighty-six. He is dying of cancer of the bowel that has spread to other sites in his body. His physician has referred him and his immediate family to the local hospice program. Mr. Hayes has had surgery and chemotherapy in previous years, but his cancer recurred, and now it appears terminal within six months.

Mr. Hayes lives with his son, Arthur, age sixty-five, a retired merchant seaman. Arthur is a widower with two sisters who live in town. Ethel, age sixty, is a married homemaker. She and her electrician husband Harvey, sixty-two, have three grown children. Sue, age fifty-eight, is divorced, and she and her daughter Roseann, age thirty, are in business together as hair stylists and cosmeticians.

Mr. Hayes has asked Arthur to look into hospice care on his behalf. Accordingly, Arthur has gone to the hospice office and is now talking to Gordon Murray, the staff social worker.

"How may we help you, Mr. Hayes?" asked Mr. Murray.

"My old Dad is dying. Doc Kerr has told Dad that he may only have six months to live. He doesn't want to go into a nursing home, and I'd like to take him home. Doc Kerr says that you can help us, but we don't know anything about it. Dad asked me to come and see what you do," said Mr. Arthur Hayes.

"Sure, Mr. Hayes. Probably the most important thing to start with is that we are primarily a medical program. Our main purpose is the relief of pain so that people who are dying can have as good a quality of life as possible," said Mr. Murray.

"The idea is to spare pain, rather than to prolong life?" asked Mr. Hayes.

"That's exactly what we try to do, Mr. Hayes. Of course, we don't try to shorten life. We just don't take superhuman measures to prolong it after it is clear that these measures would not result in any good quality of life," explained Mr. Murray.

"I have to ask about the money. I'm retired, and Dad doesn't have much beyond his Social Security. I need to know whether we can afford it," said Mr. Hayes.

"Money's not a requirement, but we do file for any insurance benefits that are available. Does your father have any health insurance beyond Medicare?" asked Mr. Murray.

"He's got a group policy from the Vesuvius. I got good rates on it, since it covers me, too, now that I'm retired. I brought a copy of the policy with me," answered Mr. Hayes, handing over the policy.

"The Vesuvius is a good, old-line company. You've got one of their Medicare supplement policies here and I think that you're pretty well covered. We accept whatever Medicare and any supplemental insurance pays. In this community, any difference between what the patient's insurance pays and the cost of care is made up from the United Fund. We have a local insurance firm that takes care of our paperwork for us, and I'll just photocopy your policy and they'll check it out, but I think that I'm on pretty safe ground in assuring you that money won't be a problem," said Mr. Murray.

"I don't want you to think that money is the most important thing, here, Mr. Murray, but Dad's sickness has been expensive, even with the insurance and our savings. You can't help but worry what's next," said Mr. Hayes.

"Sure. It's hard not to worry about it, Mr. Hayes. It's something you need to know about."

"So, how does this work?" asked Mr. Hayes.

"If you and your father want us to help, we'll come to visit you and we'll explain to him that our purpose is to keep him comfortable and free from pain. If he wants our service, and you are willing to take care of him during his illness, then the next thing we'll need to do is to determine the amount of medication he'll need to remain pain-free and yet be able to take part in the things that are going on around him. Our doctor, Dr. Gilbert, will see him and will talk to Dr. Kerr about his condition. After that, Dr. Gilbert will take care of him," said Mr. Murray.

"You mean we won't be going to Dr. Kerr any more?" asked Mr. Hayes.

"You may, but Dr. Kerr has asked Dr. Gilbert to handle this aspect of your father's treatment. It's similar to what it would be if Dr. Kerr had referred your father to any specialist. Of course, if you want to see Dr. Kerr, you may call him at any time, but the active management of your father's treatment would be in Dr. Gilbert's hands. You and your father may want to meet Dr. Gilbert before you decide anything. I think you both will like him," said Mr. Murray.

"But will I know enough to take care of Dad?" asked Mr. Hayes. "After all, I'm basically a sailor, not a nurse!"

"We can give you a lot of help. We have nurses who will visit regularly and we have volunteers who will come in and relieve you so that you can get out of the house regularly. I'll visit you weekly at least, and so will Dr. Gilbert. You won't be alone in caring for your father. And, during bad spells, we can care for your father in Wright Memorial Hospital. We have an arrangement with them and they hold a small ward for us to use when it's needed," said Mr. Murray.

"But most of the time he'll be at home, right?" asked Mr. Hayes.

"Sure, Mr. Hayes. I need to ask if there are other members of the family that can help, too," said Mr. Murray.

"Well, yes. My sisters, Ethel and Sue, live in town. Ethel's kids are grown and she's willing to help. Sue's willing, but she and her daughter run a beauty shop and she may not have much time to give, but she and Roseann, her daughter, will do their part. We're all behind Dad," said Mr. Hayes.

"He's lucky to have children who love him," said Mr. Murray.

"Dad's always been there when we needed him. I guess it's our turn," said Mr. Hayes.

"I wish everybody felt that way, Mr. Hayes," said Mr. Murray.

"OK, I'll pass this on to Dad and I'll call you. I think maybe we can manage with this kind of help. I know it won't be easy, but I think I owe it to Dad to try."

Here we have another family—not a traditional nuclear one, but a family nonetheless—that can be described as an open system. The family system appears to work very well. The elder Mr. Hayes wants to spend the last months of his life with his family and the family is willing to accept the tasks that are involved. With support from the hospice staff, we would expect that Mr. Hayes will be able to maintain a meaningful life up to his death. Obviously, with a disunited, hostile family, the outcome would probably be quite different.

Summary

In these examples, we have examined a number of issues in working with the families of older people. We have reaffirmed our contention that the older person should be treated as a valued customer and not as an object whose fate is entirely in the hands of others.

For most older people, the family (in any form) remains an important support system, both psychologically and financially. We think that the family structure is less important than the actual way in which the family functions. Those families that are open and growing are generally more supportive to older relatives than those that are closed and preoccupied only with their own current concerns.

It is also important for the professional to note the role of the older person in the family. Generally, the less integrated the older member is, the less supportive the family will be. The importance of this commonsense observation lies in the recognition that helping professionals have to accept the family very much as it is, and cannot realistically expect to markedly change relationships unless the family is experiencing a great deal of discontent with the present state of affairs.

The Benson family provides a look at the potentially harmful effects of a lack of family communication on intergenerational relationships. Also illustrated was the healthy use of reminiscence by an older person who is coming to terms with her life and trying to make sense of it. Further, Mrs. Benson's moves toward starting over represent an increasing mastery over her life. Many older people make similar moves, although, of course, they do not have Mrs. Benson's money.

In the case of Mr. and Mrs. Phillips, we see an example of a family that is much closer and more supportive of each other. While there will be considerable sacrifice on the part of all three of them, they are willing to commit themselves to a mutually supportive course of action that is constructive to the personalities involved.

The same can be said for the Hayes family. It will not be easy, but because the family system functions well and is open to the experiences of life, Mr. Hayes' life will not lose its meaning as a consequence of a lack of family support.

10

Working with Groups

In previous chapters, we have discussed working with individual persons and with their families around specific problems of individuals. In this chapter, we will look at the use of groups as a method of providing services to older persons or to their relatives.

The Nature of Human Groups

The term *group* is much abused. In recent times, there has been a tendency to use the term to describe any collective set of individuals, even when they have no shared social relationship. For example, it is not an uncommon experience to attend a convention or other large meeting and to hear a leader instruct a crowd to "divide into small groups, but try to get in a group where you don't know anybody." We are not trying to be pedantic about this, but a group in which nobody knows anyone else is not a group at all! The essence of group life is some degree of shared intimacy. Members of groups are people who, in fact, know each other fairly well, or who will come to do so if they remain in the group. Of course, a new member may not be well acquainted with the older members at first, but he or she will become integrated into the group eventually, or will never become a genuine group member. When a new group is formed deliberately, one of the problems that must be gotten through is the difficulty of any significant group interaction until the members begin to develop some kind of bond among themselves.

For the purposes of our discussion here, we will stipulate what we mean by a group. There are several elements that must be present.

1. Obviously, there must be two or more people!
2. There must be a reason for belonging that has some degree of *importance*. There is something at stake that matters to the members, even if it seems trivial to an outsider.

3. There must be some degree of *interaction* over some relatively extended amount of time. We hedge our definition with the word *relatively* since there are some kinds of group experiences that are short by plan. Most of the time, however, group interaction is something that will continue for weeks, months, and even years.

4. There is some degree of *intimacy*, however slight, that is manifested through gestures and symbols. By intimacy, we mean some amount of emotional involvement—which may not always be friendly but is nevertheless important. The necessity for an emotional bond requires some face-to-face contact, although absent members may be able to maintain meaningful contact for long periods of time, provided that there is some opportunity to renew the intimacy.

We intend here to distinguish groups from audiences and other sets of people who come together but who interact very little, and who have little or no stake in what happens over time. There are many important nongroup events in our lives, and we do not mean to imply that only group life is worthwhile. People do have significant audience experiences—concerts, motion pictures, plays, or athletic events are examples—that may be life enriching and personally important. We do not intend to minimize their value. Our point is simply that group participation is different from other social activities.

Types of Groups

There are a number of ways of conceptualizing types of groups (see, for example, Garvin, 1981 or Brieland, Costin, and Atherton, 1985). We will not review them all here, but we will list the types of groups that we think are most likely to be of use in working with older people. All of them possess the qualities of importance, interaction, and intimacy to some degree, although all types—and all groups within types for that matter—do not possess these qualities in even amounts.

There are other characteristics of groups that vary. Some groups are formal. They may have officers, a constitution or a set of by-laws, definite meeting times, rules, and minutes. Some formal groups may lack some of these features, but will have other formal structures and procedures (see the "quality circle" under the heading "Work Groups" below). Others have no formal organization at all, but operate on a highly informal basis. Some groups have a definite leader, while others seem virtually leaderless or have a kind of shared leadership. Some groups have been deliberately formed, either by the potential membership or by some parent institution. Others just occur spontaneously.

We have classified the groups that we think are most likely to involve older people into five categories. We will discuss working with some of these groups later on in the chapter.

Recreational Groups

Some groups are formed primarily to meet a recreational purpose. These groups may or may not have a formally designated leader. Frequently they are composed of people who have simply found each other through an informal process and have continued to associate because they like each other and their common activity. While there are many social gains to membership, the bonds that hold the group together are not usually deep or intimate, although one is often surprised by the degree of intimacy that has developed in some of these groups. One of the authors knows of a bridge club that has persisted for over fifty years. The members do not usually have face-to-face meetings except over the bridge table and they do not usually exchange confidential communications. Yet everyone knows when one of the members is ill or troubled, and tries to temper their interactions accordingly. Flowers may be sent if a member is ill or in the hospital, and one or more members will visit. When a child of one of the members marries, the group will buy a suitable gift. When a spouse dies, the members will attend the wake or visitation and go to the funeral. The widow can count on the other members of the group for a certain level of continuing emotional support. The intimacy that has developed over the years has provided a great deal of warmth for the members, even though the group's purpose is clearly recreational and the group has no formal organization.

Some recreational groups have, of course, a more formal structure. There is a designated leader. The activities are more structured, and there is usually some skill involved. However, learning the skill is not as important as doing it, which provides the basis for group activity. As an example, one of the authors knows a number of people who are involved in a senior swim group. The group employs an instructor on an hourly basis and meets frequently. The instructor helps the members improve their techniques, but the group does not provide basic instruction. All the members know how to swim and have done so for many years. There is a president and a treasurer, even though there are no extended formal discussion meetings. The level of intimacy is much lower than that of the bridge club, but there is a degree of it, and there is shared interaction over time. Obviously, the activity is important enough for the members to pay the instructor's fee.

Some would describe the above groups as *friendship* groups. We have chosen to avoid that term because we think that all groups develop what we prefer to call intimacy, which includes friendship, but is not limited to it. These two examples are groups that have occurred spontaneously, but recreational groups are often deliberately formed. A class that is organized primarily on an interest basis—an aerobics class in an adult education program, for example—might blossom into a genuine group over time and develop the three qualities of importance, interaction, and intimacy that would, to our way of thinking, mark the essence of group life.

Task or Work Groups

These groups are organized around a definite task or project of interest to the members. A task group may be in existence for a few weeks, or it may last over several years. In these groups, the task is central, but in order to carry it out, interaction is necessary and some degree of intimacy develops as people work together.

It is easy to confuse task groups with committees. We would like to preserve a distinction. Committees, as one wag has said, are the devil's way of preventing decision making! While committees are more or less task oriented, and they certainly need interaction, they generally lack genuine intimacy, although we must grudgingly admit that on rare occasions some degree of intimacy does develop and a committee may come close to resembling a group. Usually, however, intimacy is neither desired nor does it occur. What is more likely is that the committee will be composed of small, informal caucuses that interact with each other to achieve their separate agendas.

Some work groups are formal and deliberate. An example of this is the quality circle used in industry. Although the team that meets to discuss common problems of the workplace is organized by management and is a modern management tool, it is certainly a group because the subject is of interest to the members, there is interaction, and a certain level of intimacy is shared, although it may or may not involve friendship.

Other work groups are quite informal. One of the authors used to live in a neighborhood that, through a complicated arrangement, owned a swimming pool. Maintenance of the pool was done by a more or less consistent group of people that managed to keep the pool running for over thirty years with little discernible organization. Although it may be hard to believe, a degree of intimacy developed among the members. Somehow, the group interaction was such that the abilities of each member were appreciated while his or her weaknesses were compensated for by someone else's strengths. In other words, the members made allowances for each other—and this is an important aspect of group intimacy.

Personal Development Groups

These are groups that have as the central purpose the development of some characteristic or ability other than pure recreation. Included here are groups in which one learns a practically useful skill. Learning to speak French, Oriental cooking, or assertiveness training are examples. The difference between these groups and pure recreational groups is that the member is interested in developing skills that enhance his or her ability to cope with important life tasks that go beyond sheer enjoyment. There are, admittedly, some gray areas. We used a swimming group as an example of a recreation group earlier in this discussion. If the group were learning life-saving techniques, we would consider it a personal development group, because it aims at producing a skill that has implications beyond one's own immediate pleasure in the activity. The potential use for others seems to be an important distinguishing characteristic.

Small, intimate classes often become groups. If the class is too large for a genuine emotional closeness to develop, the members remain an audience.

Social Purpose Groups

We gave some thought to calling these groups *special interest* groups, but decided that this term has acquired such a negative connotation that we had to find another one. What we have in mind are those groups that identify themselves with a specific public problem and organize efforts to convince the public of the worthwhileness of some specific course of action. It may be that the group supports a current policy and aims to keep it before the public, or it may be that the group has an alternative to a present policy that it wants the public to adopt. An example of a social purpose group would be a local organization of older people. This group might support the continuation of current policies in the community that it believes are in the interests of older persons, and offer alternatives to current policies that it believes are inadequate. While it may be argued that this group is merely a lobbying group for the selfish interests of older persons, we prefer to regard it as a group that stands for positions that are in the public interest. This group might be linked to other local groups through an umbrella organization—the American Association of Retired Persons (AARP), for example. However, the national AARP is not a group, in our view, because a national organization lacks the intimacy necessary to genuine group life.

What distinguishes these groups from others is the emphasis on a social purpose that goes beyond the immediate interest of the members and has implications for public policy.

Therapeutic Groups

Our definition of a therapeutic group is broader than those usually given in discussions of group therapy. We include here both those groups that are sponsored by therapeutic institutions and staffed by professionals and groups that are usually called "self-help" groups. We think that they both have a therapeutic or curative purpose, regardless of the sponsorship. Therefore, we would include deliberate therapy groups sponsored by a mental health clinic in this category, but we would also include here groups for widows and widowers, for example, that have no professional direction. We lump them together because both types of groups try to help the members deal with a personal problem and get on with the business of living. The differing sponsorship does not alter the fact that both kinds of groups have a restorative or curative purpose. They only differ in method of approach to the problem under consideration.

The Role of Groups in the Helping Process

We did not use the popular term *support group* in the discussion above because we contend that all groups—as we have used the term—are support groups or they are not groups at all. People who share in the important activity of the group, interact with other members, and develop some degree of intimacy receive some amount of support from the group. The ability to recognize the role of group participation in the lives of older people can be of great assistance in the helping process. Further, skill in working with groups can facilitate the group's tendency to provide support and mutual aid to its members.

Group Work

Deliberate work with groups has grown out of several fields. Most readers of this book will have been exposed to the history of group work. For those who have not, Garvin (1981) has an excellent brief summary. Here, we only will sketch the general background. The roots lie in the settlement houses of the late nineteenth century and the Young Men's Christian Association movement. The settlements and the Ys provided two things that supported the growth of an organized approach to group life. First, they provided places to meet and engage in interaction. Second, they provided the institutional support for group leadership to develop. In many cases, the personnel of the institutions provided actual leadership, but the goal has always been to develop the leadership capabilities of the group's members and to gradually restrict the role of the professional group worker to that of facilitator or enabler.

Over time, group-serving agencies learned a great deal from those who engaged in the more formal study of what has come to be called group dynamics. The grafting on of the knowledge gained from observation and formal experiments with groups gradually formed the intellectual basis for the professionalization of group work.

As we said earlier, not all groups are formally organized with clearly identifiable structures and organizational formats. And most groups operate without professional help. In the subsequent discussion, we will distinguish between these two conditions, but we want to stress that both kinds of groups are important in people's lives and both offer the potential for support and mutual aid. Professionally assisted groups are not morally superior—or inferior—to groups that are not assisted. They are different, though, and the difference must be kept in mind when thinking about them in the context of offering help to aging persons.

Mr. Mazzelli and the Rose Club

Mr. Mazzelli is a retired grocer and a resident of the Hillsdale Retirement Center, a nursing home that includes both intermediate and skilled care. Mr. Mazzelli is not in bad health, other than some arthritis in the joints. However, he is past eighty and he didn't want to keep house for himself after his wife died, nor did he want to move in with any of his children, so he moved into Hillsdale. He has no relatives living in the city, but he does receive periodic visits from his son Guido, who is a priest in Ohio. Mr. Mazzelli's daughters, Rosa, Carlotta, and

Maria are married and live in New York, Quebec, and Texas. The nearest relative is his son Stefano, who is a manager for the regional grocery chain that bought Mr. Mazzelli's store at a price beyond his wildest avaricious dreams. Stefano was all for the sale, since he saw possibilities in the chain that he didn't think would exist if Mazzelli's Market remained independent. One of the staff nurses from the intermediate care wing has stopped to chat with Mr. Mazzelli as he sits on the back patio of the retirement center.

"Well, Mr. Mazzelli, and how are you this morning?"

"Fine, Mrs. Bennett," said Mr. Mazzelli automatically.

"We surely have had lovely weather this spring," said Mrs. Bennett.

"Yes," said Mr. Mazzelli.

Mrs. Bennett noticed a certain sadness in his voice.

"Anything wrong, Mr. Mazzelli?" she asked.

"No," answered Mr. Mazzelli.

"And how are the children?" Mrs. Bennett was fishing for a clue because she believed that something *was* troubling Mr. Mazzelli, who normally had a positive outlook on life.

"They're fine. Had a letter from Rosa yesterday and talked to Stefano last week."

"I expect that you miss them," said Mrs. Bennett, still fishing.

"Sometimes I do, but mostly I don't," replied Mr. Mazzelli.

"Oh?" responded Mrs. Bennett.

"You ever raise five children, Mrs. Bennett?"

"No, the Lord only blessed me with two, Mr. Mazzelli."

"Frankly, the best years that my wife and I had came after the last one was gone! Oh, we loved them—and they loved us—but the quiet and the freedom was wonderful. Until Gina died." Mr. Mazzelli looked down at his hands slightly gnarled with arthritis.

Mrs. Bennett waited patiently for Mr. Mazzelli to speak. She avoided saying conventional things, and being a good Catholic herself, she respected the importance of death to people who had come to grips with it.

"You know what I really am thinking about?" said Mr. Mazzelli after a pause.

"No. Tell me," said Mrs. Bennett.

"The rose club."

"The rose club?"

"Well, that's what we called it. It wasn't really a club with officers and stuff. Just six or seven of us that raised roses. We met each other at the nursery. Got acquainted and began to drop around and look at each other's roses. Used to get together at someone's house and pick each other's brains about rose culture."

"And where are they now?" asked Mrs. Bennett.

"Well, Charlie's dead, God rest his soul. Pete King lives over in Carter's Springs with his sister, worse luck for him! But Clive Nelson, Burt Stein, and Harold Nakimoto still live here and I think they have recruited one or two younger fellows. I kind of dropped out after Gina died and my hands got painful."

"And the roses meant a lot to you?" asked Mrs. Bennett.

"Well, yeah. The roses and the fellows. Roses were Gina's favorite flower, you know. She got me my first bush when we bought the first house on Granville Street. We named our eldest daughter Rosa, you know."

"Why don't you give one of your gang a call?" asked Mrs. Bennett.

"Oh, it's been four or five years since I raised roses. I expect they've forgotten me by now."

"Maybe so," said Mrs. Bennett. "Well, I've got to get back to the sick, Mr. Mazzelli. There's just one question I wanted to ask."

"What's that?"

"Why are you thinking of this now?"

"It's early spring. Good time to plant roses."

"Oh sure, why didn't I think of that?"

"You don't plant roses," Mr. Mazzelli said, managing a smile.

About two weeks later, Mr. Mazzelli had a visitor.

"Burt? What in hell are you doing here?"

"Looking for you, you miserable wretch," said a small, bald man with a big smile.

The two men hugged each other and pounded one another on the back.

"Clive and Harold are in the car. Come on out. I want you to meet a couple of the new kids in the club. They're only in their sixties, but they may come along as they mature. Ready to do some work?"

"Burt, I haven't done any work in years—and what the hell are you talking about anyway?"

As they walked out to the parking lot, Burt Stein explained. "We got a call from the director of Hillsdale. She wanted to know if there was any chance that we would be interested in giving them a hand. Seems they want to put in a small rose garden out back in the picnic area. They are paying for the bushes, but they talked us into doing the labor. We talked it over and decided we'd use their offer as an excuse to do some experimenting."

"Uh-huh," grunted Mr. Mazzelli, sniffing the air.

"What's the matter, Angelo?"

"I think I see some nosy meddling in this business."

"What's the problem? They need some simple decorative bushes, and we need the space. Our own yards are full of stuff, and we were looking for a chance like this."

"And I suppose you think I can help, at my age and with my hands like this?" said Mr. Mazzelli.

"Sure I do. Your head and your experience aren't bent, are they? Unless you'd rather not associate with the cheap help?"

"Burt, did you ever take a shot in the mouth from an old man with arthritis?"

The two men embraced again, and Mr. Mazzelli and Mr. Stein walked arm in arm out to the parking lot. As they passed the entrance to the intermediate care wing, Mr. Mazzelli stopped. Sighting Mrs. Bennett, he excused himself to Mr. Stein for a minute and stepped into the ward.

"This is your doing, isn't it?" he asked Mrs. Bennett.

"Well, sort of. The director really did want to do something with the park area, but couldn't see how it could be done without spending a lot of money. Then I thought of your rose club. That's all there was to it."

"How'd you know I wouldn't think that you were a patronizing, manipulating old . . ."

"Instinct, Mr. Mazzelli. You're just not that kind of bear."

"Well, I'll not complain this time, but next time you meddle in my affairs, I'll turn you in!"

"Sure, you will, Mr. Mazzelli. Now will you please go and play with your friends? I've got meds to pass."

Discussion

We can see that this situation will work out well. And we must ask your indulgence if we use more good examples than we do bad ones. Our belief is that if one works at it, there will be more good experiences in working with the aged than he or she might suppose.

In this example, there are several points that we want to stress. The first is that Mrs. Bennett displayed a number of qualities that are important in working with people. She treated Mr. Mazzelli as an adult, not as an old child. She was able to listen for Mr. Mazzelli's wants and did not simply pressure him into an existing activity program, as we have seen some retirement center personnel do. It's true that she took a chance in telephoning Mr. Stein and involving the rose club. But her instincts were on the side of the consumer. Rarely will one go wrong when he or she is making it possible for the consumer to get what he or she wants, although it can happen.

The most important thing about this example is that Mrs. Bennett recognized the significance that groups have for people. Although Mr. Mazzelli had dropped out of the group, he had not really left it emotionally. While the rose club wasn't a formally constituted group, it clearly embodied the qualities of importance, interaction, and intimacy. The members derived support from the group's activity and they engaged in mutual aid.

Although this was not a therapy group, activity in it had a therapeutic effect on the members. It is important for those who work with the aged to recognize the value that groups of this sort have for their members and to support participation in them. We know of an operator of a nursing home, for example, who goes to great pains to be sure that those residents who are able continue participation in community groups. This is extra work for the nursing home operator. However, the added dimension that it appears to give to the residents' lives justifies the effort.

Not all group life generates the warmth and support of the rose club. Nevertheless, group involvement is still important. Let us show you a more formal group as it engages in planning an annual event. This group meets in a senior citizens' center. The center serves a neighborhood that the City Recreation and Park Authority (known officially as CRPA, but unofficially as CRAPA in the neighborhood) defines as "working class tending to poor."

The Silver Circle

The Silver Circle Club is composed of a mixed bag of older people who have opted for membership in what may be rather loosely described as a social purpose group. The group's stated purpose is "to improve the conditions, and hence the image of the neighborhood, in the eyes of the community." The members are mostly long-time residents of the community, but there are newcomers who have gradually been accepted into the group. The center is financed jointly by the United Way and CRPA, but it is an uneasy cooperation. A group worker on the staff of the senior citizens' center meets with the group.

This is not the place to review all the theoretical bases of group work. An admirable attempt was made by Roberts and Northen (1976) and the reader is referred to their work. In this instance, the group worker, Mr. Rogers, sees himself as having the dual roles of enabler and mediator. A pleasant young man, he good-naturedly endures his colleagues' reference to the area as "Mr. Rogers' Neighborhood."

The meeting tonight has to do with the preliminary planning for the annual neighborhood fair. Each year, the Silver Circle takes on the formidable task of sponsoring a street fair designed to build neighborhood pride and to be a public relations event that will better the view that the city takes of the neighborhood. The fair has been held for several years now and, although it has had its ups and downs, somehow the event works. At least it persists. Let's go inside the meeting room and take a seat in the back. Although the official membership of the Silver Circle is nearly fifty, only eighteen people are in the room. The president is Mr. Karl Schmidt, who retired from the Findlay Tool Works two years ago. Findlay Tools is the biggest employer in the neighborhood, and many of the members of the Silver Circle Club are former employees. Mr. Schmidt was elected president of the club on the strength of his experience in the union at the Works.

Mr. Schmidt is seated at a table in the front of the room. Beside him sits Maude Fletcher, the club secretary. Pauline Moore, the treasurer, and Bertha Connolly, the vice-president, are the only members seated in the front row. Mr. Rogers sits three rows back, on the end of a row by himself.

"If you've all had enough coffee and doughnuts, let's get started," says Mr. Schmidt, as he taps his gavel on the table.

"Does anybody want the minutes of the last meeting read?" he asks.

"Move we dispense with the reading of the minutes," says a voice from the center of the group.

"Second," mumble several people.

"Hearing no objection, the minutes will stand approved as printed. Very well, let's get to the business of the street fair. I'll call on the chairmen for reports."

"Point of order, Mr. President!"

"Yes, Mrs. Gill?"

A slender, grey-haired woman rises in the second row. "Most of the people who head the committees are women," Martha Gill says in a quiet voice, "and, in fact, most of the members of the club are women. Don't you think it's time that you stopped calling everybody a chairman?"

"Uh, well, I guess it's just habit. I sure don't want to antagonize the ladies, God bless 'em."

"You already have," murmurs someone.

"This isn't the first time this has come up, Mr. Schmidt," continues Martha Gill.

"So what do you want me to say, *Ms.* Gill? Do I have to use chair*person?*"

"Why not just try 'chair,' Mr. Schmidt?" suggests Ms. Gill.

"All right." Mr. Schmidt surrenders with bad grace. "Let's hear the reports from the 'chairs.' Let's start with publicity. Mr. Cavan?"

A small, pink, rabbity man with a snow-white mustache looks up. "Yes?"

"Can you give us a report?" asks Mr. Schmidt patiently.

"No," says the little man, looking pinker than usual.

There is silence in the room.

"Is there a problem?" asks Mr. Schmidt.

"Not really," answers Mr. Cavan.

"Well, can you give us some idea of where we are in publicizing the fair?"

"Well, I've done some preliminary thinking," says Mr. Cavan.

"But you haven't yet called a meeting of your committee?"

"Well, no."

"Don't you think we ought to be starting to get something done?"

"Well, Mr. President, the fair is three months off, and I just haven't had time to get started."

"What in hell else have you got to do?" asks Ben Elston, a large, burly man.

"I've got a lot of things to do," sniffs Mr. Cavan. His mustache actually seems to twitch.

"Bunch of crap, if you ask me!" says Mr. Elston.

"Nobody did, did they?" murmurs someone.

"Who said that?" demands Mr. Elston. No one answers.

"Mr. President?" says Mr. Rogers.

"Yes, Mr. Rogers?" says Mr. Schmidt.

"I have to take some responsibility for the delay. CRPA has a new public relations person on its staff. She hasn't had time to actually get her feet on the ground, and I suggested that Mr. Cavan might want to give her a chance to get settled in before approaching her for technical assistance."

"I see," says Mr. Schmidt, "well, we'll pass on for now. Can we expect a report next time, Mr. Cavan?"

"I hope so," says Mr. Cavan, "I do appreciate your assistance Mr. Rogers."

But Mr. Cavan doesn't look very appreciative. Further, Mr. Rogers notices Mr. Elston giving him a sly look. Mr. Rogers is clearly uncomfortable, but he believes that he has headed off a potentially ugly scene.

"Next, let's hear from Mrs. Bowen on the arrangements," says Mr. Schmidt, with a bright, artificial smile.

A slim, white-haired woman with beautiful skin the color of coffee stands up. "I've talked to all the merchants in the three blocks that we'll be using for the fair. They have agreed to having the street blocked off as long as we don't block the entrance to their shops. The mayor's office will see to it that the street department will provide the necessary barricades, and the police will handle the traffic and provide security. I think that's pretty much everything," concludes Mrs. Bowen.

"Very nice, Mrs. Bowen," says Mr. Schmidt, as if to a child who has done well.

"I wish the old . . . darling would stop acting so patronizingly surprised when a black person does anything," whispers Mrs. Bowen to her husband.

"Yassuh, he shore ought to know that us black folks just loves to put on shows," whispers her husband, widening his eyes.

"Stop that, you old goat!" smiles Mrs. Bowen, giving her husband a dig in the ribs. "It's not really funny."

"I know it," Mr. Bowen replies, "but Schmidt is Schmidt, and he's come a long way."

"You're being charitable, as usual, Fred," whispers Mrs. Bowen, "but his attitude is the reason that so few blacks have been active in the group."

"You're right, as usual, Alice. We'll have to see to it that he sees some more black faces at the next meeting after the fair. That'll be the election," says Mr. Bowen looking thoughtful.

"Now, Mrs. Hammond, how about the prizes?" continues Mr. Schmidt, turning to an attractive woman whose clothing, while not new, is well chosen and carefully maintained.

"I've gotten commitments for a few, Mr. Schmidt," says Mrs. Hammond, rising to her feet.

"Please tell us about them," says Mr. Schmidt, as he gives her what he conceives of as an intimate smile.

"Look at the old fool," says Mr. Elston in a whisper to Mr. Rogers. "He's been trying to get next to Marge Hammond for years. Thinks his chances are improved since her husband died last June. She's got too much class."

Mr. Rogers says nothing, but appears to be focusing on Mrs. Hammond's report.

"Well," says Mrs. Hammond, "Mr. Elliott has promised us a ham and some merchandise certificates from the supermarket. Dixie van Ness says that she will give us a blender from the hardware, and I think that we can get some sheets and pillowcases from Porter's downtown. I have a complete list."

Mrs. Hammond opens her purse and takes out a typewritten list that she hands to the secretary, Maude Fletcher.

"Thank you, Mrs. Hammond. I'm sure I speak for all of us when I say that we appreciate the wonderful job you are doing," says Mr. Schmidt, grinning at her.

"Thank you," says Mrs. Hammond, who gives Maude Fletcher a meaningful look.

Ms. Fletcher winks at Mrs. Hammond, aware that Marge Hammond has no romantic interest in Mr. Schmidt. These public displays of unwanted interest *were* embarrassing.

In the next half-hour, a lengthy report is given by Bertha Connolly, the vice-president, on the cultural events, displays, sales, and contests that are planned for the fair. We'll skip Ms. Connolly's report and move to the last item on the agenda. Each year, the street fair clears three or four thousand dollars from entry fees, sales of "white elephants" and craft items, and raffles. The raffles are of questionable legality, but they have been going on so long that the police and the district attorney close their eyes to them on the grounds that a good cause is being served. The problem that always arises concerns the latter point. What is the good cause this year?

"Well, folks, that just about wraps it up for now as far as the fair is concerned," says Mr. Schmidt. "Now, how will we spend the money?"

Mr. Elston ponderously rises to his feet. "Well, Mr. President, I have an idea. We could use the money to purchase the materials to build some attractive planters for the shopping area of our neighborhood. We could put some small trees and shrubs in the planters and maybe attach some permanent concrete benches to them so people could rest when they come to shop. Lots of our people still use our local stores because of the convenience. If we can keep the shopping area attractive, maybe the stores will do well enough that they won't lose all of their customers to the shopping malls."

Mrs. Hammond rises and says, "That's a good suggestion, Mr. Elston, but I wonder if it is what we should be doing. There are so many needs that are important. I have recently become interested in the new shelter for abandoned children. This shelter is in the old Hunkler mansion downtown. They need furniture and bedding. While the shelter is outside the neighborhood, we have to recognize that many of the children who will use it will come from the neighborhood."

Mark Bates, who had said nothing during the meeting so far, stands up and says, "I think that the Silver Circle should use the money in the neighborhood, but I am not drawn to the planters and benches. I doubt if we could build very many with the funds that will be available."

"We could make a start," says Mr. Elston, rising. "And next year we could build some more and so on until the project is finished."

"But this would commit the group to a long-term project. We've never done that before," comments Mr. Cavan, sensing that he has an ally in Mr. Bates.

"That doesn't mean anything, Cavan," says Mr. Elston.

"I think we might discuss Mrs. Hammond's suggestion," says Mr. Schmidt.

"You would," snarls Mr. Elston.

"What's that supposed to mean?" asks Mr. Schmidt, whose face is beginning to get red.

"Haw, haw!" says Mr. Elston.

There is more discussion. Each idea attracts a core of supporters, and the meeting begins to bring out additional hostility.

Finally, Mrs. Gill speaks up. "Could you give us some help, Mr. Rogers?"

Everyone turns to Mr. Rogers. He feels uncomfortable with the attention, but, he reminds himself, this sort of thing is why he is here.

"You all have done very well in planning the street fair," says Mr. Rogers as he rises from his seat. "It's a very ambitious undertaking, and it means a lot of hard work for everyone. I can see that spending the money is as difficult as making it."

There are a few smiles, but most people wait for some kind of a resolution to the problem.

"The easy thing to do would be for Mr. Schmidt to appoint a committee to prepare a proposal. That, of course, would only delay action, and it might not suit anybody anyway," thinks Mr. Rogers out loud. "One way to proceed would be to consider both Mr. Elston's and Mrs. Hammond's ideas, while keeping the options open for one or more alternatives. As I understand it, we're talking about at least three and maybe four thousand dollars."

"We took in $3,765.86 exactly last year," says Ms. Moore, the treasurer, looking up from her ledger.

"Mr. Elston, how much would one planter and bench combination cost?"

"It's not cheap, but I've got some friends who are cement masons and they tell me they can build one of these things for about $800, donating some of the labor."

"Would any of the merchants be willing to contribute something toward this project?" asks Mr. Rogers.

"I dunno. Maybe. I could ask. What do you have in mind?"

"I was thinking that the club might be able to assist the merchants in taking some interest in improving the shopping district. Suppose we approach the merchants, offering to design the planters and benches. Further, we could offer to build one or two as demonstrations. If the merchants like the idea, then the long-term aspects of the project could be done jointly without involving all the street fair's profits."

"Say, that's not a bad idea," says Mr. Elston.

"If you want, I'll be glad to go with you to the Neighborhood Merchants Association meeting to sound them out," says Mr. Rogers.

"First, let's talk to some of them individually, Mr. Rogers. I don't think it's good tactics to spring it on them at a meeting," says Mr. Elston.

"Will this meet with everyone's approval?" asks Mr. Rogers.

There is a general murmur of assent.

"Does anyone have an objection?" asks Mr. Schmidt.

No one objects.

"Now, does this mean that we won't do anything about the shelter?" asks Mrs. Hammond.

"Well, what I was thinking was that we could identify some specific furniture and buy it. Maybe we could talk to the people at the center, get a 'wish' list, and identify some articles within the budget. We might want to consider taking on the center as an ongoing project," suggests Mr. Rogers.

"All right, I would be willing to talk to the center director about the matter. I know we can't do everything with a small amount of money," says Mrs. Hammond.

"On the other hand, Mrs. Hammond, we can use our money and our talent to spotlight neighborhood and community needs. This may help direct the attention of other groups to these needs. In short, the Silver Circle can be a real catalyst for helping the community to address some real problems," says Mr. Rogers.

"Even if we spend $1,600 on the planters and a similar amount on something for the shelter, we would have several hundred dollars left over," notes the treasurer.

"Then, maybe we ought to consider spotlighting some neighborhood problem at the next meeting," says Mr. Bates. "I like the idea of using the club's funds as spotlight grants in order to raise issues."

Again, there is a murmur of assent through the group.

"Well, we've had a good meeting tonight," says Mr. Schmidt. "Have we any more business? Is there a motion for adjournment?"

"So move," says a voice followed by a "second" from the back, so the meeting ends.

Discussion

This meeting is not intended as comic relief! There are several points that we want to make.

First, we have attended real meetings that did not differ much from this fictionalized one. We said that the official membership was nearly fifty, but that only eighteen people were in the room. In most groups, it is rare for all the members to be present. In what we have called social purpose groups, most of the work will devolve on a relatively few people. It would be nice if more were involved, but they generally will not be, except on rare occasions. This is simply a fact of life for those who work with groups. One might reason that older people would be more available for group activities, since more of them have grown children or are retired. It doesn't work that way, because older people are as occupied with activities as are younger people—unless, of course, they are frail or bedfast, and even then many are doing something of importance to them. The point is that the person who works with older people should not be discouraged when he or she finds participation rates of older people to be about the same as similar groups of younger people.

Second, there are tensions within the group. Mr. Schmidt exhibits common sexist and racist attitudes. These attitudes are resented, and Mr. Schmidt may find himself called into account at the next election of officers. True, his sexism is traditional and even unconscious and his racism is of the patronizing variety. We cannot envision Mr. Schmidt engaging in overtly hostile sexual or racial politics. However, the comparative mildness of his biases does not justify them, and we think that Ms. Gill and the Bowens are entirely justified in taking him to task.

There are also tensions between Mr. Cavan on the one hand and Mr. Elston and Mr. Schmidt on the other. It is true that Mr. Cavan is not highly efficient, and he could use some assertiveness training, but it is clear that Mr. Elston is a bully who enjoys baiting mild-mannered people and that Mr. Schmidt is one who enjoys the use of his office. Mr. Elston is not a false stereotype. There are people like him in every group, and they make life difficult for those who work with groups.

Mr. Rogers' attempt to "take some of the heat" isn't really helpful. We have seen professionals use this strategy, and it usually fails. We have found that the most successful strategy with the Mr. Elstons and Mr. Schmidts of the world involves some form of confrontation. This should not be done angrily, but it must be firm. If Mr. Elston is unable to get his way, or if no one takes his bait, he will be forced to adopt a more civil approach to relationships. Mr. Schmidt will no doubt learn at the next election that one of the dangers of office is that an autocratic leadership style is not appreciated in a voluntary association, except in extremely threatening situations when the organization's back is against the wall.

Mr. Schmidt has further endangered his reelection by his clumsy attempts to seduce Mrs. Hammond. Many group members have hidden agendas, and these may well include attempts at seduction. We are not saying that it is inappropriate or unusual for older people to be sexually interested in each other. However, in this case, Mr. Schmidt is using his office in an exploitative way, and Mrs. Hammond is clearly not interested. Mutual attraction is one thing. Seduction is quite another because it involves deception and exploitation. Although Mr. Schmidt is so clumsy he is certainly going to be unsuccessful, he still comes off as ridiculous and insulting in the eyes of other group members. Such behavior isn't admirable in people of any age.

There is little that helping professionals can do directly about hidden agendas. For example, no good purpose would have been served if Mr. Rogers had gotten up and said, "Mr. Schmidt, quit trying to play up to Mrs. Hammond and get on with the meeting." Most hidden agendas have to do with power, and are usually less obvious than Mr. Schmidt's. The most effective thing one can do is to keep the group's focus on the real issues before them while publicly ignoring the hidden agendas.

We want to make one other point. Mr. Rogers did earn his money by the way he used his skills in working out the conflict over spending the proceeds from the street fair. He listened to each proposal, suggesting a way in which Mr. Elston, Mrs. Hammond, and Mr. Bates all won something and nobody lost everything. Not only that, but he turned the group's attention to its stated purpose of involving the neighborhood in self-improvement.

Further, he did not take over the group. He waited until he was asked for a suggestion, and he got out of the way when Mr. Schmidt exercised the legitimate role of his office. Although we have simplified the group process for reasons of space, this description is not unrealistic. We have seen skilled professionals bring groups together using this approach. Alan Filley, whose field is business management, has stressed the importance of following win-win strategies in group decision making (Filley, 1975). While no side gets everything (as one side would in a win-lose situation), both sides get something of what they want, neither loses face, and group cohesiveness is enhanced. As simple as this technique is, we have seen it work regularly. This was, indeed, a good meeting.

The Therapy Group

Before we leave the subject of using groups, we want to briefly show you one more type—the therapy group.

We have argued that the essence of group life lies in having an activity of importance, a fair amount of personal interaction, and some degree of intimacy. It is easy to understand the importance of these characteristics in most groups, particularly those in which people have a long history of membership and a great investment in time, energy, and effort. The therapy group is generally a "formed" group. That is, an agency, clinic, hospital, or individual therapist has brought the members together in order to provide a group treatment experience that will be of value to the participants. Despite the apparent artificiality of the group's formation (group members rarely are known to each other before the therapeutic experience), the therapy group, in time, acquires the basic characteristics of group life. In the therapy group, the activity is important for its therapeutic effect. Personal interaction is generally short—sessions are usually limited to an hour or two—but can be intense. The degree of intimacy varies with the nature of the condition for which treatment is offered, but most people will develop at least some degree of "we" feeling over time.

There are a number of approaches to group therapy, some more directive than others. As a general rule, the more self-directed that the members of the therapy group are, the less directive the therapist needs to be—or can be, for that matter. Conversely, the less motivated and the more withdrawn and remote the group members, the more likely that the therapeutic approach will take on a more directive tone.

The group that we will show you below is mainly composed of persons who are fairly well self-directed. The members are widows or widowers over sixty who have experienced some degree of clinical depression. Some of the members have been treated as inpatients in the psychiatric ward of the local general hospital. They are still being followed as outpatients. Others have been treated primarily as outpatients by psychiatrists in the community who are on the hospital's staff. The therapist is Walter Meers. Mr. Meers is unusual, but not unique, since he has both a Bachelor of Science in Nursing, with a specialty in psychiatric nursing, and a Master of Social Work. He has also had additional training in working with groups.

When one of the local psychiatrists has a patient that he or she believes could benefit from the group, a referral is made to Mr. Meers, who is also on the hospital staff. If, in consultation, Mr. Meers and the psychiatrist agree that the patient will probably benefit, the doctor advises his or her patient of the availability of the group. The patient is encouraged to have an initial interview with Mr. Meers. If, after this interview, the patient and Mr. Meers agree that the group experience is of potential benefit, the patient is invited to the next group meeting.

Attendance is voluntary, of course, and each member is told that he or she will not be "dumped" as a patient if he or she is not accepted into the group or does not choose to participate in it.

There is a fair amount of turnover in the group's membership, as most patients are able to regain their balance and get on with their lives. Some patients simply drop out, finding that the group does not meet their expectations after all.

This Tuesday night, a new member is coming to her first meeting. Currently, the group has eight members, and the new patient will be the ninth member. Mr. Meers seldom accepts more than ten people in the group at any one time, preferring to refer potential members to other therapists when he judges that the group is large enough. The group meets at the hospital in a room that is about the size of an ordinary living room. There are comfortable chairs, two small couches, some accessory tables, and, against one wall, a long table on which stands a coffee maker and a small refrigerator. The room is lit by a combination of floor and table lamps instead of the usual institutional ceiling fluorescent fixtures.

Mr. Meers has asked Mrs. Isaacs, the new member, to come a few minutes early. As the other members come to the group meeting, Mr. Meers introduces each of them to Mrs. Isaacs. As we enter the room to observe, we find the the entire group seated. Some are drinking coffee or a soft drink.

Mrs. Able, who is seated next to Mrs. Isaacs, asks, "So how long has it been, Mrs. Isaacs?"

"Three weeks," says Mrs. Isaacs with a polite smile.

"Would you like some coffee, Mrs. Isaacs?" asks Mrs. Holmes, who sits on Mrs. Isaacs' other side.

"No, thank you," replies Mrs. Isaacs.

"Were you in the hospital?" asks Mrs. Able.

"Yes, for two weeks. I just got out a few days ago," answers Mrs. Isaacs. She begins to make hand-washing motions and looks toward Mr. Meers, who is watching her. He smiles at her, and she manages to smile back faintly. Then she begins to cry softly.

Ms. Dale gets up and comes over to stand behind Mrs. Isaacs' chair. She puts her hand on Mrs. Isaacs' shoulder.

"It's all right. There's been a lot of tears shed in this room. That's one of the things that the group is for," says Ms. Dale.

"I thought I had cried all I could when Jack died," says Mrs. Isaacs, "but I still have more tears, I guess."

"Do you want to tell us about it, Mrs. Isaacs?" says Mr. Meers.

"Not now. Maybe next time, but not now," says Mrs. Isaacs.

"Whenever and if ever you want, Mrs. Isaacs," says Mr. Meers.

"It's very hard, isn't it?" asks Ms. Frankel, who, at sixty, is one of the younger members of the group.

"Well, yes, it is," smiles Mrs. Isaacs.

"And no one else can tell you to stop crying, so we won't," says Mr. Edwards, one of the two men in the group.

No one says anything for a few minutes. Mrs. Isaacs sits quietly, looking into space. Ms. Dale continues to gently pat Mrs. Isaacs' shoulder. Ms. Frankel and Mr. Edwards continue to look at her in a friendly way.

"The worst part for me was the junk," says a new voice.

"Garibaldi had nuts and bolts in little jars. He had pieces of wood stacked in the garage attic. He had several boxes of electronic stuff. He left a dozen unfinished projects behind him when he died, and every time I'd go to throw anything out, I'd get to thinking about him and I'd just sit there and cry for the longest time," says Mrs. Garibaldi.

"Have you thrown any of that stuff out now?" asks Ms. Frankel.

"Finally, I asked one of my husband's friends to come over and go through it. He sold some of it at a garage sale and took the rest to the landfill. Took me two years to get around to it," says Mrs. Garibaldi.

Mrs. Isaacs has been following the conversation despite her vacant look.

"Have you been a member of this group for two years?" she asks.

"Oh, no, Mrs. Isaacs. Only a few months. You see, I didn't get depressed right away. It was a kind of a delayed reaction, but when it came it really hit. I was upstairs for nearly a month!" says Mrs. Garibaldi.

"Did you . . ." Mrs. Isaacs began.

"It's all right to ask any question that you have, Mrs. Isaacs," says Mr. Meers.

"Well, I really don't think I should right away," says Mrs. Isaacs.

"Oh, it's all right, Hon," says Mrs. Garibaldi, smiling. "I'm out of the woods, now, and I can talk about it. What did you want to ask?"

"Well, did you feel that it . . . just wasn't worth it after your husband died?"

"I think she wants to ask if you tried to commit suicide," says Mrs. Able.

"I wouldn't have asked that," says Mrs. Isaacs, showing her annoyance at Mrs. Able.

"It's all right, Mrs. Isaacs," says Mrs. Garibaldi. "One of the things that this group does is to give us a place to 'let it all hang out' as my daughter used to say in the 1960s! One of the rules is that you can ask anything. Of course, the person you ask can simply say that he or she doesn't want to answer. In my case, I didn't try to kill myself. One day I just sat down and stopped living. My daughter found me just sitting in a chair, staring into space, and brought me to the hospital."

"And are you over your husband's death now?" asks Mrs. Isaacs.

"No. But my doctor and Mr. Meers and the group have convinced me that I am still a worthwhile person and that life is still important. I'll always miss Garibaldi, I think."

We will leave the meeting now. It looks as if Mrs. Isaacs will fit in and will find support in the group.

Discussion

Groups of this sort are not unusual. In smaller communities, however, it is unlikely that specialized groups of widows and widowers would be available. More likely, Mrs. Isaacs would find herself in a group that had a wider age range and perhaps a wider range of problems related to depression.

We didn't show Mr. Meers doing much. However, he had done more than showed during the meeting. First, he had carefully selected the group members in consultation with their doctors. This is a common practice. Some readers may wonder about those who were rejected. Isn't it undemocratic, even cruel, to fail to include people who may be hurting just as badly as those who are included?

It must be understood that therapists are not magicians. Not everyone can benefit from what a therapy group has to offer. A therapist must decide whether group membership is in the best interests of both the group and the individual patient. Inevitably, some persons will be referred to other groups or simply not encouraged to participate in group therapy. Generally, this is done because the therapist believes that he or she cannot work effectively with the person, that the person would not benefit from the group experience, or that the person might indeed be harmed by the exposure to the kind of frank exchanges that occur in group sessions. This is a professional decision. While it is sometimes difficult to exclude a person from a group, it must sometimes be done.

Mr. Meers' role in the part of the meeting that was described was limited to introducing Mrs. Isaacs and offering her support at several points in the meeting. He had also eased Mrs. Isaacs' introduction to the group by inviting her to come early. That way, she did not have to meet the whole group at once.

We had a brief glimpse of the group's process in relating to new members. This was a highly compatible group and the members were unusually able to let Mrs. Isaacs begin to relate at her own pace. No one told her how to behave or how to think. They accepted her "as is" and exhibited an easy acceptance of her and her obvious pain. Another group might have been composed of less empathic members, but careful selection has made this group a more supportive, therapeutic experience than it might have been under other circumstances.

Groups of various kinds are important parts of human life. They can be of enormous help to older persons. Helping professionals should be aware of their potential and encourage their clients and patients to maintain meaningful group contact whenever possible.

11

Community Resources

The professional in aging should attempt to help older persons secure what they want and need to live their lives satisfactorily. In some cases, material goods—food and clothing—are desired. In others, specific services, such as home health nursing and transportation, are wanted. In still others, counseling, help in cutting through bureaucratic red tape, or information about resources or strategies that might be used to solve a problem may be needed. When an older person comes to a professional for help, it is sometimes possible for the worker to secure what the older person wants through the resources available in the worker's agency. Thus, if the older person's only need or want is transportation to a physician's office twice monthly, a worker employed at an agency that provides transportation for older persons should be able to arrange appropriate services with relative ease.

Often, however, older persons have a range of wants and needs, not all of which can be satisfied through the services of the worker's employing agency. No health or social service agency can do everything and most provide a fairly restricted range of services. Human-service workers thus have the responsibility not only of helping the older persons who come to them make use of the services that their employing agencies provide, but also of helping these people find and use resources available elsewhere in the community. The purpose of the first section of this chapter is to discuss how the worker becomes knowledgeable about the range of resources available to older persons and how the worker helps the older person secure needed or wanted resources. We focus on the types of programs and services that are typically available to help older persons solve problems and the ways in which the older person and professional work together in an effort to satisfy wants and needs.

The second section of this chapter is concerned with how professionals are involved in modifying or building resource systems to better meet the needs and wants of older persons. It is not uncommon for the professional working in the field of aging to discover a number of older persons who share similar problems that are not adequately addressed by the formal resource system in the community. A worker might discover, for example, that there are a number of frail older persons who are uncomfortable staying at home alone during the day. Although they do not need skilled nursing care, they have trouble walking to the toilet or may be frequently confused. They and their families wish there were some way to find an honest, reliable person who would "sit" with them, and provide needed assistance and security for a reasonable fee. The worker may conclude that there is some need for a "sitter" referral service in the community and take steps to organize such a service or persuade others to do so.

There are also situations in which organizations of older persons, or organizations that work on behalf of older persons, seek a change in federal, state, local, agency, or corporate policy to benefit older persons. Helping professionals in the field of aging often contribute to these efforts. We give examples of how professionals in the field of aging can work to effect such changes.

Overall, the intent of this chapter is to help the reader become familiar with the kind of helping that extends beyond the bounds of the agency or organization for which he or she works. While not all helping professionals may be in a position to spend much on-the-job time creating new resources or changing laws or policies to improve the lives of older persons, it is our position that the direct service worker can contribute to these processes in important ways. Thus, we discuss both leadership and support roles in large-scale efforts to improve community life for the old.

Becoming Acquainted with Community Resources

One of the first things a professional should do after taking a new job is to become as familiar as possible with the resources available in the surrounding area. The best place to start is in one's own agency. While some agencies provide formal orientation to agency functioning, the new employee frequently must take the initiative if he or she is to learn quickly the details about all the programs and services the agency provides. One can begin by reading official documents (brochures, program descriptions, policy manuals), but this kind of activity should be supplemented by keeping one's eyes and ears open, by getting to know other members of the staff, and by asking questions. In any organization some policies are more flexibly applied than others, and some fellow staff members are more cooperative than others. If the agency serves a wide variety of persons, some staff members may be more interested in serving aged persons than others. It is important for the worker to develop a "mental roadmap" of his or her agency, which serves as a guide to the services the agency is prepared to offer, the criteria used to determine who gets what services, and the policies or personalities that might serve as barriers to responding quickly and with a minimum of fuss to needs or wants of older persons. It is important to remember that orientation to one's own agency is a continuous process. Staff turnover, changes in funding patterns, and changes in program guidelines are common phenomena in health and social service agencies. Thus, one must work hard (particularly if one is employed in a large organization) to keep up with resources available to those one serves.

Equally important is knowing where to go outside one's employing organization to find resources. The complexity of this task varies as a function of the size of the community in which one is working. In a community of five thousand people that is not near a major population center, a newly employed worker should be able to learn quickly the names and locations of organizations that provide formal services to older persons, the extent of the services, and the criteria used to determine who is eligible for the services. Such an undertaking is virtually impossible for one person in a large city working alone, even if he or she devotes full time to it.

Fortunately, in most localities of moderate size one does not have to start from scratch. Usually, some agency has the responsibility for providing information and referral services for the community. In larger communities there is often a special information and referral service for the elderly. One of the functions of information and referral services is to maintain an up-to-date listing of formal services in the community. Every so often, these agencies publish a resource guide that contains agency names, addresses, telephone numbers, and a description of services and eligibility criteria.

The newly employed professional is well advised to get the most recent edition of all such local guides and keep them handy for reference. They can be a good beginning in becoming familiar with community resources. An effective professional, however, will use them only as a guide. As noted above, staff and programs change, usually too fast for any printed guide to keep up with them. Also, guides for public distribution can never be sufficiently detailed to include nuances in policy, or the information about who in a given agency is cooperative and who isn't. This knowledge is essential to the person who wants to give good service to the aged.

As a result, an effective worker will develop a personal information and referral guide. It will be based on the printed guide, but supplemented by information gleaned from contact with other professionals, responses from older persons who have used (or tried to use) other agencies' services, and one's personal experiences with other resources. Some workers keep this information in their heads, but a more typical approach is to develop a series of file cards, available for easy telephone reference. In one's personal guide one can note the names of staff at other agencies who provide the most prompt and effective help. One should also make note of restrictions on services (for example, transportation to residents living west of Main Street only; closed all day Thursday) and special services that the agency has provided in the past or that one has provided to that agency. (As is discussed later, when one is asking a colleague for a favor, it may sometimes help to remind that colleague of favors you have done for him or her in the past.) Before long, the file-card system of keeping track of resources is likely to be obsolete. As personal computers make their way to human service professionals' desks, workers will likely find that they can acquire computerized versions of official resource guides that they can easily modify and update with personal notes and information.

Formal Resources

The range of services available to older persons in a community varies with the size of the community and the community's interest and ability to fund services. Generally, a large and prosperous community is likely to have more services available to its older citizens than a smaller, less prosperous community. In the following section, we describe some resources available to older persons regardless of where they live, as well as other formal resources that may also be available, particularly in more densely populated areas.

Social Security

Programs administered by the Social Security Administration provide substantial financial support to older persons, as was discussed in detail in chapter 3. Each locality in the nation is served by a Social Security office that older persons must contact for information about social security retirement, disability, and survivor's benefits, Supplemental Security Income, and Medicare. Human service workers should become familiar with their local Social Security offices. In sparsely populated areas, Social Security workers meet on a regular basis with potential beneficiaries near their homes. One can help an older person save a great deal of time and expense by knowing when and where claims representatives are available for consultation. In many instances, arrangements are made for Social Security representatives to meet with beneficiaries in places where older persons gather, for example, congregate nutrition sites and senior centers, either to provide individual consultation or to answer questions in a group setting.

Public Welfare

Each state has a department of public welfare that typically has offices at the county level. The services offered to older persons through the department of public welfare vary considerably from state to state. They may include financial assistance in addition to SSI, food stamps, emergency assistance, home health programs, case management, volunteer assistance, and transportation. In states with adult protective service laws, social workers at the public welfare office investigate cases of suspected abuse and neglect of older persons and make pertinent recommendations. While most services offered through public welfare departments are aimed at low-income persons, protective services are typically available regardless of socioeconomic status. Those who work with older persons should become familiar with the specific services offered by their local public welfare agencies, the criteria for eligibility, and the ways that those needing the services can gain access to them.

Agencies on Aging

In 1965, Congress passed the Older Americans Act in an attempt to address the needs of all older (sixty-plus) persons, regardless of income. With federal assistance, localities have developed area agencies on aging (AAAs) whose job is to assess needs of local older persons, set priorities for service development, coordinate existing services, and stimulate the orderly development of needed new services. Area agencies on aging have varying geographic service locations. In most places they serve a number of counties, but some states have a single AAA, and in some places an AAA may serve a single city or county.

Few area agencies on aging offer services other than information and referral directly to older persons. They have, however, been instrumental in establishing new services (e.g., congregate nutrition, transportation) and in providing a focal point within the community for raising issues related to services to the aged. The professional in aging should become familiar with the area agency on aging in his or her locality and the services that are affiliated with it. Frequently, the AAA can be the catalyst for developing new programs to meet older persons' needs within a community.

Community Mental Health Centers

Beginning in 1963, federal funding became available to encourage localities to develop community mental health centers. These centers, which frequently serve a fairly large geographic area, provide a wide variety of mental health services to persons of all ages. A high proportion of the clients served are persons formerly institutionalized for mental health problems. They include elderly or near-elderly persons who were in mental hospitals for many years. Community mental health centers are expected to not only help those who have been hospitalized, but also to provide services that will prevent mental illness. Thus, they can be an important resource for persons whose problems are not severe enough to require hospitalization. Because mental health centers typically operate on a sliding scale fee system, they can be particularly helpful to low-income older persons who cannot afford private therapy. Services vary from mental health center to mental health center, but may include individual or group counseling, case management, day treatment, and emergency services.

In many communities, the mental health center provides a twenty-four-hour crisis line that individuals are encouraged to call if they are contemplating suicide or are experiencing other emotional difficulties.

Public Health Departments

Public health departments serve virtually all areas of the nation. Much of their work involves prevention of the transmission of communicable diseases (which includes giving immunizations), environmental health, and services to mothers and children. Services available vary widely from state to state. Some public health departments run special clinics for the elderly, focusing on screening and treatment for hypertension and other chronic illnesses. In some areas they are able to provide home health care services for the elderly and disabled. A professional who provides services to the elderly is well advised to learn about services available to older persons through the local health department.

The services of the agencies described in the previous section are funded, either entirely or to a large degree, through the federal government, and are generally available throughout the United States. In many areas, additional services are available that are funded with federal, state, local and/or private monies. The kinds of services to be described next may be administered by a wide variety of agencies, and some may not be available in a particular community. The professional trying to familiarize him- or herself with a new community should inquire about the availability of these services.

Nutrition Services

In the last two decades, area agencies on aging have been successful in developing congregate nutrition services for older persons. Although these services do not exist in every community, they can be found in many small towns and rural communities, as well as in urban areas. Nutritious noon meals are served in a local facility (community center, church hall), and anyone sixty or older, regardless of income, is eligible to participate. The purpose of these programs is not only to help ensure an adequate diet for older persons, but also to provide opportunities for social contact and recreation. Participants also gain information about nutrition, health, and other available services. There is no formal charge for the meals, but participants are encouraged to make a daily donation to help defray costs. These services are particularly helpful to low-income older adults who live alone, and sites are often located in areas where high concentrations of low-income elders reside.

Another important nutrition service is home-delivered meals. Some home-delivered meals are available as an extension of the congregate meals program, although churches and other voluntary community agencies may also provide this service. Both chronically disabled adults and those recovering at home from an acute illness or surgery find these services helpful. Often, a physician's recommendation is necessary for a person to receive home-delivered meals. The cost can range from nothing to the full cost of the meal.

In many communities low-income elderly persons can take advantage of Department of Agriculture surplus commodities distribution programs. Having been certified as eligible, one can come to a food distribution site and pick up an allotment of butter, cheese, milk, or other food products. The kinds of commodities distributed through these programs have varied in recent years, depending upon agricultural surpluses.

Transportation

Transportation is often a major problem for older persons. Some have never learned to drive an automobile, others are prevented from doing so because of health problems, and others cannot afford to maintain a vehicle for themselves. As a result, many communities have developed special transportation programs for the elderly, often using Older Americans Act funds available through area agencies on aging. Minivan service that will take older persons from their homes to congregate nutrition sites, physicians' offices, grocery shopping, and to other services is often available. In some places, the vans are equipped with hydraulic lifts for those who are wheelchair-bound or have difficulty walking. In some areas, volunteer driver services have been organized to help older persons with transportation needs. These services are particularly useful for persons located in isolated, rural areas.

In urban areas, mass transportation is often cheaper for the elderly during nonpeak hours. Some public transportation systems have adapted certain vehicles to accommodate persons who have trouble climbing stairs.

Recreation

Many local park and recreation departments run special programs designed specifically for older persons. These include sports, exercise and fitness programs (swimming, bowling leagues), tours and trips, dances, and musical groups. Senior centers (discussed below) provide a variety of recreational activities for elders. Some older persons prefer to make use of recreation services developed especially for their age group, while others participate in programming that is not age specific.

Volunteer Opportunities

A number of programs coordinate the use of senior volunteers. Perhaps the best known is the Retired Senior Volunteer Program. Available in many communities of moderate and large size, this program helps match seniors interested in doing volunteer work with community agencies seeking volunteers. In many cases, transportation to the volunteer work site is provided for those who wish it.

In some communities SCORE (Service Corps of Retired Executives) matches retired professionals with small businesses that can use business advice.

The Foster Grandparents Program is also available in many communities. The intent of this program is to pair older persons with developmentally disabled or neglected children. Although listed here as a volunteer program, Foster Grandparents is geared toward low income elders and provides modest compensation for older persons who work with children. Similarly, the Senior Companions program provides a small stipend to low-income older persons who assist with long-term care of disabled elderly persons in hospitals, nursing homes, or at home.

Many health and social service organizations recruit and train volunteers of all ages. Some older persons interested in volunteering approach the agency in which they are interested directly. The programs described in this section are special in that they are geared exclusively toward older adults and try to find the best match between the older person's interests and the community agencies seeking volunteers.

Education

In many communities, special educational services are offered to seniors. Sometimes there are special seniors-only classes offered through the public schools' community life education programs on topics ranging from playing the guitar to genealogy. Classes may focus on "aging" issues (health education, wills, and trusts) or on topics of general interest.

A number of colleges and universities offer regular college courses to seniors for no cost or reduced tuition. Courses may be applied toward a degree or may be taken on a noncredit basis. Some junior and community colleges have been particularly successful in recruiting seniors and include a social as well as an educational component in their programming.

A wide variety of educational experiences is available throughout the world through the Elderhostel Program. Colleges and universities host short (usually one to two weeks) programs that bring older persons to their campuses for coursework, local tours, and social activities. The hostelers live in the college dormitories, eat in the cafeterias, and take several short courses designed especially for them. Seniors interested in Elderhostel programs apply through a national office and pay transportation and program fees themselves.

In recent years, hospitals have become increasingly interested in providing health education courses and programs for older persons. They may provide free or low-cost courses on topics ranging from "Living with Arthritis" to weight reduction. Some supplement courses with membership programs, offering free periodic health screening, discounts on drugs and other products, and a simplified admissions process should hospitalization become necessary.

Multipurpose senior centers often provide a wide range of short courses and other educational opportunities, geared specifically to the interests of their participants.

Employment

Many elders seek full- or part-time employment. While seniors may make use, like anyone else, of state employment service offices, there are also several programs targeted specifically at older workers. We have already discussed the Senior Companions and Foster Grandparents programs as volunteer programs that pay small stipends to older persons. These two programs are funded through the federal ACTION program. Another series of programs is funded through the Department of Labor under the Senior Community Service Employment Program. Project Green Thumb employs low-income retired farmers and agricultural workers in tasks involving community beautification, horticulture, and soil conservation. The Senior Aides Program places older workers in community service organizations, and pays a small stipend.

Protective Services/Abuse Prevention

Those working in the field of aging sometimes encounter elders in need of protection from themselves or others. In most states, the legal responsibility for investigating situations where the need for protective services is suspected is the public welfare department. Two types of situations are most common. One involves an older person, usually living alone, who is thought to be not physically and/or mentally competent to provide for his or her own health and safety. A protective service agency will assess such a situation and make a recommendation about the validity of allegations and whether services should be offered or legal action taken. In extreme cases, a sheltered living arrangement and/or legal arrangements to manage the older person's finances appropriately are made through court action. More often, less extreme measures are taken that protective service workers believe will improve the living situation of the older person without diminishing his or her freedom.

The other type of situation that calls for protective services action is where abuse or neglect of an older person by a relative or other caretaker is suspected. Abuse and neglect take many forms, including physical assault, verbal and psychological abuse, neglect of the care of frail and bedridden persons, theft or extortion of finances or property, and unnecessary institutionalization. Many states have mandatory reporting laws that require professionals to report cases of suspected abuse and neglect to a designated state agency. The protective service worker investigates allegations of maltreatment. If the allegations are found to be accurate, the worker acts as an advocate for the abused or neglected older person. Interventions may include counseling for the abuser and abused, introduction of services (homemaker, home health aide) to the home, temporary respite care for the older person, removal of the older person from the abusive or neglectful environment, and criminal prosecution of the abuser. Legal assistance may be sought in protective service cases to help the older person understand her or his rights and to secure restitution of resources taken from the older person by the abuser.

Older persons most at risk for abuse and neglect are those with severe physical problems and/or mental illness that results in confusion and irrational behavior. Many suffer from Alzheimer's disease. Recent attention to the problem of elder abuse has focused on prevention programs aimed at family care givers. The hope is that if care givers receive education about Alzheimer's and other debilitating conditions and learn some techniques for easing their own burdens in caring for elders, they will be less likely to strike out in anger, and the incidence of abuse will be decreased. Professionals should be aware of education and support groups for care givers in their communities and refer families at risk for abuse to these resources.

Housing

The various types of housing available to older persons are discussed at length in chapter 6. Professionals should learn about the housing options available to the aged in the communities where they work. Some larger cities provide housing referral services for the elderly. Such services have information not only about the housing choices available for older persons, but also about individuals who are interested in sharing their homes with elderly persons in exchange for fees or services.

Senior Centers

In many communities, the focal point for services for the elderly is a multipurpose senior center. Senior centers vary considerably in the range of programs and services they offer. Centers almost always provide a facility where seniors can gather for activities, classes, or just to chat with other seniors. Most provide noon meals in conjunction with the Administration on Aging's congregate nutrition program. For many older persons, senior centers are an important source of social activities, mental stimulation, and access to resources. A wide variety of services may also be available that reduce older persons' needs to call or visit other community agencies.

Center personnel are usually well-informed about senior services throughout the community. An older person with a problem or concern can usually learn from a professional at the center which agency is most likely to be helpful. This information and referral function of senior centers can save the older person a great deal of time and energy in resolving a problem. In addition, many senior centers schedule regular times when participants can meet with representatives of community agencies. Thus, Social Security representatives, food stamp workers, public health nurses, mental health workers, and public welfare workers may have regularly scheduled times when they are available to consult with seniors at the center. Since most centers provide transportation to and from the center, it is possible for an older woman without a car to visit with her friends at the center, enjoy a nutritious noon meal, confer with a Social Security representative, and have her blood pressure checked all on the same day at the same place without having to arrange any special transportation.

Membership Organizations

Mass-membership organizations are also important resources for older persons. Many seniors are active members of local chapters, and others benefit from programs and services without being locally active.

The largest and best-known membership organization for older persons is the American Association of Retired Persons (AARP). With over 27 million members over age fifty, this organization provides a wide range of services and programs. For a nominal membership fee, members receive a monthly magazine, access to a low-cost mail-order prescription drug service, discounts on products and services, and the opportunity to participate in a variety of education and service programs. These include preretirement education, services to the recently widowed, consumer protection and education, defensive driving, and education about insurance. AARP is also a powerful lobbying group that advocates for older persons at the state and national levels.

Other national membership organizations for older persons include the National Council of Senior Citizens, the National Association of Retired Federal Employees, and the Gray Panthers. Specific programs and activities vary from locality to locality.

Long-Term Care

The kinds of services that can be helpful when an older person needs long-term care are discussed in chapter 12. These are important community resources, and the professional should be well-informed about them.

Legal Assistance

In many areas, legal service programs designed specifically for the elderly are available. They are often funded through the Older Americans Act. Also available to the elderly are legal services designed for low-income persons. Legal service programs provide advice and consultation by an attorney or paralegal personnel concerning problems including divorce, guardianship, eligibility for programs, wills, and consumer fraud. Legal representation may also be provided. Legal service personnel may also take an advocacy stance by publishing guides to legal issues and speaking before groups of older persons to help them understand their rights. The professional who encounters an older person with legal problems should refer that person to a private attorney or to a local legal services office.

How to Make a Referral to Another Service Agency

Because few agencies provide all of the services an older person might need, service personnel often find they must refer a person with whom they are working to another agency to get the service he or she wants. The procedures used for referrals may vary, depending on agency policy, the capabilities of the older person with whom one is working, and the urgency of the situation.

In some cases, it will be enough to give the older person the name and telephone number of the agency likely to be able to help with the problem. One would normally take this approach with a person who is self-confident and well accustomed to weaving her or his way through bureaucracies. To follow up on the effectiveness of the referral, one might ask the individual a week or so later if he or she has gotten in touch with the suggested agency and whether an appropriate service has been arranged.

In other cases, the service provider would take a more active role. Suppose, for example, that an older woman who is concerned about her invalid sister calls a senior center's social worker. The woman knows she needs some help in caring for her sister, but is not able to state precisely what kind of help she would like because she is unfamiliar with the available services. The only reason she called the senior center is that she had participated in an educational program there some years ago and heard that "there is someone at the senior center who will try to help older people with family problems." After talking on the telephone with the woman, the social worker might arrange a home visit to assess the situation and determine what services might be most helpful. At the home visit with the sisters, the social worker would explore the services available in the community, how often the services are likely to be available, the eligibility criteria, and information about how to pay for the services. If, on the basis of the interview, the social worker believed that the sisters might have some trouble arranging for the services themselves, he or she might ask them if they would like arrangements to be initiated for the service. With their permission, the social worker would then contact agencies providing appropriate services (for example, homemaker, home health care, transportation), discuss the sisters' situation, and make plans for services to begin. Having made these referrals, the social worker would subsequently talk to the sisters and the agencies to find out whether the services were being delivered satisfactorily. The social worker's role in referring the sisters ends at the point where he or she is satisfied that they are receiving the agreed-upon services.

In still other cases, the human service worker might be working with older persons in need of a wide range of services to maintain themselves in their own homes. In chapter 12, we discuss the professional's role as case manager in long-term care. As case manager for an infirm older person, the professional not only makes referrals to appropriate community resources, but also works cooperatively with the older person and the numerous agencies involved. The professional actually coordinates the services and serves as the point of contact if there is a change in the older person's needs or if there is any question or confusion about the services to be provided.

Less Formal Resources

Formal resource systems, while very helpful, by no means represent all of the resources that a professional might call upon to help older persons. Some needs and wants do not fit neatly into the categories of services provided by agencies. Some organizations and individuals are ready to provide limited and specialized help, but the availability of their resources is not widely known.

In one community we know of, an anonymous donor regularly replenishes an emergency fund that is administered by a local clergyman. Social service personnel can apply for funds on behalf of their clients, and the clergyman decides whether he can appropriately provide the money. Social service workers understand that the fund can be used only if no other resources are available. This system of old-fashioned philanthropy may offend some because it categorizes some of the needy as deserving and others as undeserving. All the same, those who work with the aged should be aware of any such arrangements in their communities, since they can provide the solution to some older persons' problems. It is also important to realize that if one goes to such a source too often or for problems that are perceived as trivial, the source may no longer be available.

Other resources may be more public but severely limited. Fraternal organizations, for example, may have a policy of paying for medical supplies for members within their geographic area. Thus, it may be useful to know whether the person with whom one is working is a member of such an organization.

In most communities there are many clubs and organizations whose goals include the duty to improve life for citizens in the community. Persons who work with the aging are often able to call upon such groups in particular situations. For example, a low-income older woman is snowed in following a heavy blizzard and cannot get to her physician for an important visit. She calls a social worker for help about what to do. The social worker thinks immediately of a young friend who told her he had been elected president of his fraternity at a local college. Within hours, two young men have cleared the older woman's sidewalk of snow, enjoyed coffee and cookies in her kitchen, and have performed a community service project.

Similarly, organizations can often be approached for funds to meet a specific older person's need. Many have funds set aside for philanthropic purposes. The professional with a contact among Rotarians, Civitans, or Elks, for example, can often make a successful case for a club to help pay for a low-income older man's dentures or for a plane ticket so that an older woman can attend the funeral of her only sister.

If one is judicious, one can often arrange for free or reduced charges for services from local merchants or professionals. If one becomes known in the community as someone who asks for favors rarely and wisely and only on behalf of people who need help and are unable to get it from conventional sources, one is likely to discover that people are more generous and helpful than one might have expected. In most communities there are not only physicians, attorneys, and dentists who will provide services for free or at reduced cost on occasion, but also plumbers, exterminators, mechanics, and funeral directors.

The key to using these informal resources is personal contact and one's reputation in the community. This is why professionals who grew up in a community or have had considerable experience in it can often be more successful in securing resources for the people with whom they work than can newcomers. To work well outside of the formal service system means one must know a wide range of types of people. Contacts made through involvement in a civic club, a church, a PTA, or through work with a youth organization can be invaluable in securing services.

Also, the ability to successfully ask for favors depends, in part, on one's willingness to give them. Human service personnel should be prepared to assist others when they can, with the thought that the help will probably be reciprocated in the future. Thus, if you are asked to speak at the local high school or at a civic club, or if an acquaintance inquires at a ballgame about whether his mother might be eligible for your agency's services, it is best to respond promptly and cooperatively. Particularly in a small community where one is known as a service provider, it is important to recognize that in some sense one is "on the job" twenty-four hours a day. The impersonal bureaucrat who attempts to rigidly separate personal from professional life is not likely to be successful in developing and using informal resources for the benefit of those he or she serves.

Modifying Programs or Developing New Programs

Thus far we have talked about how the professional gets to know existing programs and services in the agency and community and how the professional mobilizes these resources on clients' behalf. Many professionals, however, not only use what is currently available, but also work to modify and improve the local service system for their older clients. This can involve changing policies and programs within their own agency, adding programs to the array of services their agency offers, or working with others in the community to develop a new service.

Developing Resources within One's Agency

While there may be a temptation to leave program development in the hands of agency executives and planners, in fact, professionals who work directly with consumers are often in the best position to identify problems with services and to suggest new services. Many excellent ideas for service innovation come from direct service workers, and we believe that agencies should involve those closest to the consumer in planning for change. The amount of involvement an individual professional is likely to have in program development will depend on that professional's job description and the climate of the agency and community. At the very least, human service personnel should know how program change typically evolves and be prepared to participate in the process.

Changes in an agency's programs may be contemplated when there is dissatisfaction with the way the programs are currently working, when there is a perception that the agency could respond to an unmet need, or when funds become available. Often, the change process begins informally as several staff persons find themselves talking about how current programs could be improved or about new services the agency could offer. As the ideas are discussed more fully, the staff members who first began talking about them may explore their feasibility with other staff members and with their supervisors. If the ideas continue to sound promising, an individual or group takes responsibility for putting the proposed innovations in writing.

This process involves stating clearly what is proposed and why, attempting to identify the advantages and disadvantages of implementing the change, identifying how much the innovation would cost (in time, money, and other resources), and identifying who would pay the costs.

At this stage, it may also be helpful to think about who would favor the change and who would oppose it. While many opinions are taken into account, it is important that those planning services try to find out how potential consumers of the service react to the idea. As we have noted numerous times in this text, the primary job of professionals in human services is to satisfy the needs and wants of the consumer. Programs or innovations that are planned without the advice and comments of those who are expected to use them are unlikely to be successful.

To take the example given at the beginning of this chapter, suppose a professional working at a senior center has received a number of calls about frail older persons who are uncomfortable staying at home alone during the day. Several of these older persons and their children have asked the worker to locate a sitter to be there for their safety and prepare a noon meal. With some experience in trying to find sitters, the professional has learned that no agency in the community systematically links people who want sitter service with others who want part-time employment. He has occasionally been able to find someone who will work as a sitter through his personal contacts, but just as often he has been unable to help those who call him.

It occurs to the professional that the senior center might be able to develop a sitter referral service that would assist those needing sitters and other older persons interested in employment. He begins by exploring this idea informally with his supervisor and other professionals at the center. Since they think it is a good idea, he develops a brief, written proposal that outlines his ideas about how the service might work. His colleagues suggest some modifications, and he incorporates them into the proposal. In the proposal he has estimated how much developing the service would cost in time, money, and other resources and how many people are likely to make use of it. To get potential consumer reaction, he discusses the proposal with the center's advisory committee of senior participants. He may also discuss his ideas with personnel from other agencies that serve the aged (or that refer people to employment) to see if there is any opposition or if they have any suggestions to make.

Assuming all has gone smoothly thus far, the professional, together with his supervisor, makes plans to present the proposal to the board of directors of the senior center. In most agencies all new program proposals or major program modifications are subject to board approval. He plans carefully for this meeting. He includes in his presentation information that documents the need for the service, its relationship with the center's other services, expected costs, the number of people who are likely to use the service, and his plans to evaluate whether the service is meeting its goals. He also includes information about support for developing the service from the advisory committee, colleagues within the center, and other agencies in the community. The final decision about whether the new service will be offered is made by the board. If, however, he has support from his colleagues, the advisory committee, and other community agencies (and if the board does not view the project as too costly for the agency), it is likely that the board will approve as well. The center will then have a commitment to develop the proposed service.

Of course, not all ideas for innovations within one's agency are implemented with as much ease as described in this example. Others may not think your idea is as good as you think it is. Or you may have an idea for an innovation that everyone agrees is excellent, but too costly to implement. One must be prepared for setbacks and frustration, but we believe that the good professional will always keep an eye out for opportunities to improve services.

Collaborating for Change

It is not uncommon for human service workers who work directly with the aged to be involved in collaborative activities aimed at policy change that will affect older persons. The direct service worker will not usually work in a major leadership position in policy change efforts, since these jobs usually are given to professionals with special expertise in community organization, planning, and legislative processes. At the same time, many of the major policy changes effected in the last twenty years to benefit older persons have been influenced in significant ways by the ideas and efforts of those who work most closely with the aged. The amount of time you spend in working toward policy change will depend on your job description and your agency's priorities. It may range from none to quite a bit. Some human service workers also contribute to policy change through their involvement in professional organizations and as private citizens.

A discussion of the many strategies for community change that might be used on behalf of the aged is beyond the scope of this book. Readers are referred to Ecklein (1984), Burghardt (1983), and Cox et al. (1984) for more extensive discussions. Here we shall give two examples of collaborative activity aimed at change and explain how a direct service professional might be involved.

Creating a City Commission on Elder Affairs

The directors of a number of agencies that serve older persons in a small city have begun meeting together for lunch. They realize that although their agencies have separate functions, they serve many of the same older clients. Each agency has special funding needs and funding sources, and none of them can provide all the services and programs for older persons they would like. Most appeal some time during the year to the city council for discretionary funding for special projects. In discussions with their boards of directors and citizen advisory groups, they realize that they are not only competing with the police, water and sanitation, and road departments, but also with each other for the discretionary funding the city has available. The amount of discretionary funds allocated each year for programs for seniors is unpredictable; sometimes certain agencies get none at all. Agency directors have found that long-range planning is difficult under these circumstances.

After a number of meetings, the agency heads conclude that they can be more effective in advocating for older persons for city funds if they work together than if they work separately. They decide that the city council will be more responsive to the needs of older persons in the city if a special commission were established that would respond directly to the requests of older persons and the agencies that serve them. The commission they envision would have an annual budget that would be devoted to special programs and projects serving older adults in the city. In discussions with their boards and consumer advisory groups, they have found there is considerable support for the establishment of a city commission on elder affairs. Having set for themselves the goal of establishing such a commission, each goes back to his or her staff members for ideas about how to persuade the city council that the commission should be created.

Here direct service professionals may have a number of ideas. Some may know city council members or staff personally, and may begin talking with them about establishing a commission. Others may have contacts with the news media. They may suggest that a series on the needs of older adults in the city in the local newspaper or on the local television station would bring added attention to the concerns of older persons and the need for the city to respond in an organized way. Since feature stories often work best with concrete examples, professionals with direct knowledge of, for example, older persons who need transportation services or home-delivered meals may introduce reporters to older persons willing to discuss their experiences. Some workers may also be involved in helping older persons to express their wishes directly to the city's political leaders. Those who work with groups of older persons may get their advice on how to work to create an elder affairs commission. They may encourage vocal and interested older persons to contact city officials directly to express their points of view. This may involve assisting older persons who wish help to prepare for speeches to the city council, chamber of commerce, local civic clubs, and the like, advocating the commission idea. Petitions signed by older persons favoring the commission may also be influential. Those who work directly with older persons can help them organize to develop petitions and obtain signatures of as many seniors as they can get. Public hearings may be scheduled on the commission idea, and workers can often assist with transportation and with helping seniors who wish assistance to prepare testimony about the need for better, more comprehensive services.

It should be obvious that an effort of this kind can require the work of many people, including sympathetic persons in city government, agency executives, boards of directors, consumer advisory groups, and older persons themselves. In many cases, the essential linkage among these is the direct service worker. This person can provide his or her agency director with information about unmet service needs and about individual older persons willing to take on leadership roles in the policy change effort. In this way, the professional who is primarily involved in daily contact with older persons can contribute substantially to a large-scale change effort that will have long-term effects on the city's willingness to take responsibility for older persons' concerns and needs.

Improving Services for Abused and Neglected Elders

Another way that the professional in daily contact with older persons can contribute to policy changes is through work with professional organizations. We encourage those working with older persons to become active in the professional organizations appropriate for their professional training (e.g., National Association of Social Workers, National League of Nurses) and in their state and local organizations that work on behalf of older persons. Many states now have state gerontological societies that have regular meetings to exchange information about the aging process and about providing services to help people age successfully. A state gerontological society meeting is an excellent place for professionals to get new ideas about service provision and about proposed or recently enacted policy changes that affect older persons. It can also be a place where concerned professionals and older persons organize to advocate for a specific policy change.

Let us suppose that a number of professionals who work with older persons in a given state are concerned about the situation of older persons who are abused or neglected. Although the state recently enacted laws establishing protective services for older adults, professionals who investigate complaints find that few resources are available to help the older persons found to be abused or neglected. Since shelter or foster homes are in short supply, the only place in many communities to house an older person who should be removed from an abusive environment is in a nursing home or mental hospital. Severely understaffed agencies are charged with the responsibility of counseling abused and abuser, as well as trying to prevent abuse in the community.

One approach to seeking ways to ease this situation is working through a state gerontological society. Program meeting organizers (who include direct service professionals) have decided that prevention of elder abuse and the establishment of better services for the abused should be a major theme of their annual meeting. By selecting this as the theme, they hope to draw the attention of the public and of state legislators to the need for increased funding and services to deal with the problem.

In planning for the annual meeting, organizers think of several ways that they can highlight the need for better services. They begin by making a special point of seeking the help of professionals who have direct contact with older persons who have been abused or neglected. A special session is developed where workers are encouraged to present case examples (properly disguised to maintain confidentiality) that will highlight the need for improved services. They invite a speaker from another state where services are better developed to discuss how the need for better services was documented, how appropriate funding for the services was secured, and how the services were developed and implemented. They also invite members of the state legislature and policymakers in major state agencies to respond to the issues to be presented. They may prepare a resolution that they think is likely to be adopted by the society membership, favoring more state funding and specific legislation for services for abused elders.

It should be clear from this example that direct service professionals concerned about abused and neglected elders are participating actively in efforts aimed at major policy change. They serve on the program committee for the annual meeting and are involved in providing the basic information needed to influence policymakers. After the annual meeting is over, they are likely to be involved on various committees seeking to influence legislators and state agency personnel. Many are likely to testify at hearings in the state capital when legislation to improve services is considered. This level of involvement is apt to require the active support of their employing agencies, since it will involve time away from normal job responsibilities. An agency interested in improving services, however, will very likely support this activity and adjust the professional's schedule accordingly, since it is in the agency's long-range interest to have the legislation enacted. If successful, the policy change efforts will benefit both the agency and the older adults it seeks to serve.

These two examples are not intended to be exhaustive in describing the ways that professionals can be involved in policy change. Workers in the field of aging work in these and many other ways to improve living conditions for older adults through influencing policy and legislation. Our point here is to help you see that promoting successful aging can involve far more than simply helping older persons take advantage of the services one's own agency currently offers. We encourage you to think about how you can be involved in large-scale change and to take advantage of opportunities for participation.

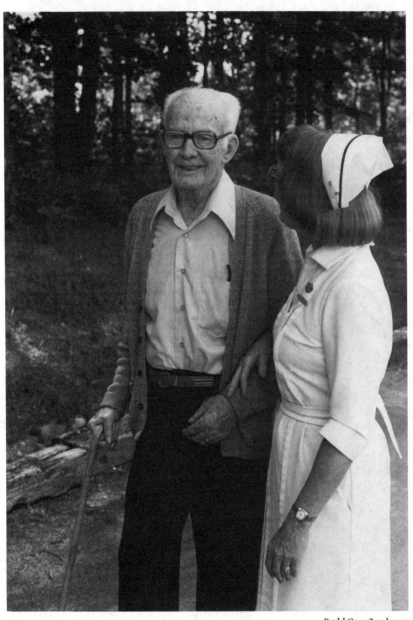

Budd Gray/Jeroboam

12

Long-Term Care

More people are living longer than ever before. In the years ahead, we expect even greater numbers and a higher proportion of the "frail elderly"—those seventy-five and over. These people are the age group most at risk of being unable to live independently. Many will need long-term care because they will have physical or mental health problems that will require continuing attention.

What Is Long-Term Care?

Long-term care refers to a variety of medical and social interventions designed to help persons with chronic illnesses and impairments live as satisfactorily as possible with their conditions. It can include medical treatment and therapies (physical therapy, speech therapy), provision of support for carrying out the activities of daily living (homemaker service, Meals on Wheels, special transportation), supportive counseling concerning loss of functioning, and coordination of services. Long-term care can be provided to a person (1) residing in a nursing home or other institution, (2) living in a normal home environment, or (3) living in supportive housing. Increasingly, professionals are involved in developing and maintaining long-term care arrangements for older persons, although much day-to-day care is provided by family members and friends, and may not involve any formal helping service.

Involvement of Service Professionals in Long-Term Care

The focus in this chapter is on how professionals can work cooperatively with family members and others in the older person's natural helping network to provide the best help with a chronic health situation. Often, this is a difficult task. The problems from which the frail elderly suffer often require continuing, daily attention, since symptoms and needs can change dramatically from day to day or week to week. Family members who want to help are often overburdened with their own commitments to work and their own families. They experience painful choices when deciding how to invest their time and their resources. Many communities have services designed to help frail elders live as successfully and as independently as they can, but often the services are poorly coordinated. Sometimes essential services are not available. Finally, long-term care services are expensive. Older persons may not receive needed care because they and/or their families are unable to afford the type of care that will promote their optimal functioning.

Because long-term care arrangements are so important in contributing to the well-being of older persons, we are devoting a special chapter to them. As a professional in the field of aging, you are likely to be involved with long-term services in one or more of several ways. If you work in a senior center, counseling agency, an acute care hospital, or a program or agency that provides long-term care services, you will find yourself helping older persons and their families assess the needs for long-term care arrangements and you will be developing plans to meet those needs. As a professional in an organization that provides long-term care for older persons in a community setting, you may find yourself as a direct provider of services or a case manager who coordinates the services of a variety of providers. Finally, you may be employed in a social service role in a nursing home or other institutional setting. Here your job will be to work with others in the facility to provide the best possible care for institutional residents and assist their family members in contributing to that care. You will help arrange for discharge of those patients who leave the institution.

This chapter will address these three types of professional roles. In each section, we illustrate the types of situations you are likely to encounter, some of the specific activities you are likely to engage in, and special issues and concerns.

Assessing the Need for Long-Term Care Services

It is important to point out that over 80 percent of long-term care services are provided by family members and close friends. Sometimes there is little involvement of professionals. We can all point to examples from our everyday lives. An older man is recovering at home after several weeks of hospitalization from a heart attack. He knows that his heart and circulatory problems are chronic and will require continuing care and attention for the rest of his life. His wife monitors and administers his prescribed medications and drives him to a physician for follow-up visits. She assists him in following the exercise routine advised by his physician and prepares meals suggested by the hospital dietitian. She talks with him when he is fearful and depressed about his limitations.

In another case, an older woman suffers from the early symptoms of Alzheimer's disease. Her somewhat younger sister, who lives with her, monitors her activities carefully. The younger sister gradually takes on primary responsibility for management of the household. She does all the driving and shopping for the two, while encouraging the older sister to do what she can for herself. She keeps a close watch, however, to be sure that the environment is safe and that she does not leave her sister alone at home. As the disease progresses, she takes on more and more responsibility. She wonders what will happen if her own health should fail or when her sister's condition will worsen to the point where she no longer can provide the needed help.

Neither of these situations is unusual. Family members want to provide help to their older members with chronic conditions. They often do so for long periods of time without assistance from the formal helping system. In some cases, the help they provide on their own is so taxing that the family members put their own health at risk. Long-term care services are typically requested at two points. First, they may be requested following a crisis (for example, hospitalization for a stroke or broken limb), when hospital social service personnel meet with the older person and his or her family to make discharge plans. Second, help is often requested when the resources of the family have been overtaxed for a long period and the situation has become desperate. In the latter circumstance, earlier intervention could have prevented the crisis. Later we will discuss how the situation could have been approached to lessen the possibility of having to plan in desperation.

When a social service professional receives a request for help in making long-term care arrangements, the first task is to assess the older person's situation. Second, it is necessary to discuss how the older person and his or her family can achieve the best possible functioning.

Among the most important tasks in the assessment process is evaluation of the current physical and/or mental health status of the older person. Here the opinions and advice of a physician and other health professionals are critical. Basic questions that need to be answered include: (1) Is health status likely to improve or deteriorate? (2) What types of rehabilitation or therapies can result in improved performance? (3) What can the older person do unassisted? (4) What can he or she do with limited assistance? A wide variety of measuring tools can be used to assist in assessing the physical and mental functioning of older persons (Kane and Kane, 1981). Hospitals, long-term care institutions, home health agencies, and others typically use one or more of these assessment instruments in developing long-term care plans. Often, personnel assist in administering these instruments and in using results to develop a long-term care plan.

If, however, you work in a program without a medical component, it is vitally important that you advise older persons and their families to begin with a comprehensive assessment of physical health and functioning. It is not uncommon for family members to decide on the basis of their own observations that an older member "needs" institutional care. Unnecessary institutional placements result when a solution that is better suited to the older person's needs may be possible.

Also important is an assessment of the older person's social functioning. Kane and Kane (1981) review a number of standardized measures of social functioning and point out that assessment of social functioning is important to the person assisting with long-term care arrangements for several reasons. Effective social functioning tends to be associated with physical and mental functioning. Those who have good social functioning have a better ability to cope with health problems and maintain autonomy. Improved social functioning is one of the goals of long-term care arrangements and thus is one of the benchmarks against which a successful long-term care plan can be assessed. Issues to be addressed in an assessment of social functioning include the older person's sense of social well-being, his or her ability to cope and adapt, and the nature and quality of his or her social relationships.

Assessing needs for long-term care also involves a careful evaluation of who is available to help the older person and what these persons' resources and limitations are. We saw the importance of this in chapter 9. It is important to know if a spouse, siblings, children and/or grandchildren are available and willing to help. What additional demands are there upon their time? Are they physically able to provide the needed care? Are they motivated to be of assistance? Will they help reliably? Sometimes family members commit themselves to tasks that are beyond their capacities. Increasingly, older persons are discharged from hospitals with complex treatment requirements, including the use of hospital equipment and the need for carefully monitored medications. If the care giver at home cannot learn to keep the equipment functioning or is unable to read well enough to follow complicated directions, the outcome can be disastrous. Similarly, some persons overestimate their ability to cope with the stress of the daily nursing care of an ill family member. The health and stamina of the proposed care giver should be assessed as long-term care arrangements are planned.

The physical environment should also be assessed. It is wise for the professional assisting with long-term care to make a home visit if care is to be provided at home. Attention should be paid to basic aspects of the physical environment. For low-income persons in rural areas, there may be questions about the availability of a telephone, the presence of electricity, indoor plumbing, or the adequacy of home heating or cooling. Are modifications necessary to accommodate a wheelchair or walker? All these factors will contribute to the appropriateness of a long-term care decision.

Other factors include the cost of the proposed arrangements and the availability of needed services within the community. Unfortunately, many of the services that would contribute to a successful community-based long-term care plan are either too costly for the older person and his or her family or are simply unavailable. The human service worker should, of course, be familiar with the array of services in the community where the older person lives (home health nursing, adult day care, home-delivered meals) and the costs of these services. He or she must be able to discuss which of the services will be covered by Medicare, Medicaid, and/or the older person's other insurance and which costs must be borne by the family.

Thus, assessment in long-term care planning involves putting together information about a variety of factors. These include the physical, mental, and social situation of the older person, the capabilities and motivations of family members and close friends, the physical environment of the older person's home, the resources available in the community, and the costs of those resources. The aim of the assessment is to describe realistic options available to the older person and his or her family.

The social service professional usually is able to offer several options. The professional can provide support and encouragement to the current care givers to help them continue doing what they have already been doing. He or she can engage one or more community resources to assist the older person and the family with homemaker services, physical therapy, transportation, or respite care within the home environment. Third, the professional can assist in placing the older person in a long-term care facility (nursing home or domiciliary) appropriate to the older person's health status and level of functioning.

Support for the Family Care Giver ──────────

In some long-term care situations, professionals work only with family members to provide them support and encouragement that helps them carry on as primary care givers for a frail elderly person. The professionals function as teachers, advisers, and sounding boards for families. In the case described above, the woman whose sister is in the early stages of Alzheimer's disease may approach a professional at a senior center to discuss her concerns about her sister's deteriorating condition. While the professional may suggest concrete services (respite care, for example), the younger woman may well refuse such services, stating that she is able to cope now, but that she is glad to know of emergency or backup help that she may request at a later point. Ideally, the professional will call her from time to time to see how she is doing and offer support. This type of activity represents the younger woman's beginning link with the formal helping system and may be all she needs at this point. What is important is that she has a contact with potential sources of help. This interaction can provide a sense of reassurance.

More formal support services for family members are also available in many communities. Support groups have been organized for families of Alzheimer's patients, of persons recovering from strokes, and of persons with other chronic conditions. These groups may take several forms. Some are self-help groups run by the members with little professional involvement. More often, professionals serve as consultants to the groups. The groups meet regularly and provide members an opportunity to share fears, concerns, and gratifications of caring for a chronically ill family member. For some people, they provide an opportunity for catharsis, since they are places where everyone shares the same types of problems. Discussion of these problems is encouraged, since it may help people find solutions. The groups also serve an educational function. A group for family members of those who have had strokes, for example, might include open discussion with a neurologist, speech therapist, or occupational therapist. Specific techniques for dealing with speech impairment or ambulation might be discussed, and literature on recovery from stroke could be available.

People who attend such meetings often report receiving encouragement and renewed stamina as they learn that they are not the only ones coping with difficult situations. Many professionals believe that this assistance can be invaluable in helping families become more resourceful care givers. The groups help them cope with frustrations in constructive ways. We mentioned in an earlier chapter that reports of elder abuse are on the rise. Research into this phenomenon (Giordano and Giordano, 1984) suggests that abusers are often overburdened care givers to chronically ill family members. Professionals believe that education about caring for impaired elders and contact with other families can help prevent elder abuse as well as put family members in touch with resources they can use when their own abilities are overtaxed.

Another resource for family members is respite care. At times, even highly committed people need a break. Perhaps they are physically or mentally exhausted with the care of an Alzheimer's patient in the home. Or perhaps a middle-aged woman caring for her ill mother wants very much to attend her daughter's wedding in a distant city, but is fearful for her mother's situation while she is gone. Many communities offer respite services—temporary, substitute care for the older person while the regular care giver is away. This is generally provided in one of two ways. In some situations a qualified sitter, with the backing of a home health care agency, will come into the home and provide the needed care. In others, a hospital or nursing home designates a number of beds as respite beds. The older person can be admitted for a temporary stay and receive qualified nursing and other needed care while the regular care giver is unavailable. Respite services are often costly and may not be covered by insurance. At the same time, they may be just what is needed to provide the regular care giver with the rest and refreshment that is necessary to resume care.

Community-Based Long-Term Care

Another situation in which professionals become involved in long-term care is through agencies that provide community-based long-term care services. A community-based system of long-term care is a coordinated effort within a geographic area to meet the health and social service needs of frail elders, making it possible for them to continue to live in their own homes. These services supplement the efforts of family members to avoid the need for institutional care. For older persons without a family care giver, they often provide the support that makes it possible for a person living alone to stay in his or her own home.

Throughout this text, we have described supportive services (home-delivered meals, home health nursing, chore service, homemaker service, specialized transportation) designed to help older persons. Generally speaking, these services have been developed rather haphazardly in most communities. A person about to be discharged from the hospital after a stroke, for example, might have to deal with four or five different agencies and intake workers to receive needed services for a period following hospitalization. It would take a very well-organized person indeed to keep track of what service is coming when, how they are to be paid, and what the services to be performed are. In most cases ill older persons (or their family members) are not so well organized that they can coordinate the various services effectively. The result, unfortunately, is that older persons find themselves going back to the hospital or into a nursing home because care in the home provided by several uncoordinated agencies is too confusing.

Recently a number of states and communities have instituted case management services to provide the coordination of long-term care services. The role of case manager is usually filled by persons trained in social work, nursing, or public health. Case management involves locating, coordinating, and monitoring a set of services. Usually, case managers serve people who remain in their own homes, but the concept can be extended to include people in specialized institutions if no other coordinating service is available. Early reports (Skellie and Coan, 1980; Taber, Anderson, and Rogers, 1980) suggested that the approach can be helpful in supporting frail elders who wish to remain in their own homes. However, Rubin and Johnson (1982) found that case managers did not focus well on the tasks of monitoring and coordinating—which are important aspects of the case manager's job. Further, recent research by Wood and Estes (1988) has found that federal budget restraints have served to limit most case management services to medically oriented agencies, since they are reimbursed by Medicaid, Medicare, or private insurance.

Case management is still in its infancy. Development of successful case management requires substantial commitment to the care of older persons within the community. Participating agencies must agree to plan cooperatively, and professionals must be free to collaborate freely with each other. Finally, participating agencies must be willing to change policies, procedures, and methods when they are clearly not to the benefit of the consumers of the service. This is much easier to say than to do, especially when there is competition for scarce resources. At this stage of the development of case management, most persons who try to help older persons with chronic conditions stay in their own homes must be prepared to "wing it" and to do their best to link the older person with appropriate services. To illustrate the way in which we think case management ought to work, we will use another example that we have written for the purpose.

Mr. Marshall

Mr. Marshall is seventy-five years old. He is still in the hospital recovering from successful coronary bypass surgery. Although recovery from the surgery is expected, Mr. Marshall is likely to need help with activities of daily living for quite some time. Mr. Marshall has been living alone. He has a forty-five-year-old unmarried son in the community who works the day shift at the candy factory, and Mr. Marshall recognizes that his son can provide him with only a limited amount of help.

With Mr. Marshall's permission, the hospital social worker has asked a case manager from a local home health care agency to stop to talk with Mr. Marshall. The case manager, Ms. Carroll, is an experienced nurse with a B.S. degree in nursing. She has some additional work toward a master's degree in public health, and she continues to plug away at her courses. Let's listen as she enters the room.

"Good morning, Mr. Marshall. I'm Connie Carroll from the Cherokee Hills Home Health Care Agency. Mr. Clark, the hospital social worker has asked me to stop to talk with you. Are you feeling up to talking about leaving the hospital?" She takes his thin, pale hand in her firm, dark brown fingers.

"You're not from around here, are you?" asks Mr. Marshall, looking at her brown face and tightly cropped hair.

"No," Ms. Carroll laughs easily, "I'm a Canadian—really, I'm from Jamaica originally, but we moved to Ottawa when I was twelve."

"Well, well," says Mr. Marshall as he leans back against his pillows.

Ms. Carroll isn't annoyed. At least, she doesn't show it. "Does it matter, Mr. Marshall?" she asks with a smile, letting the Jamaican lilt show.

"No. Not really, I guess. I just was startled, seeing a black person—I mean, I've seen black people before, but. . .," his voice trails away.

Ms. Carroll smiles warmly. "I know. We're everywhere nowadays, aren't we?"

Mr. Marshall's embarrassment passes easily because of Ms. Carroll's good humor. She is comfortable about being black, and does not allow Mr. Marshall's comments to upset or offend her.

"Well, I guess I'd better earn my pay, Mr. Marshall. Let's talk about leaving the hospital. Dr. Munson says in about a week or so, yes?"

"That's what he told me. But I'm not sure how it is going to work."

"Well, let's think about that. I know that you have one son, George, and that he is single and does not live with you. Any other family?"

"No. My wife died six years ago. I've got a brother, but he lives in

Wisconsin and all of his family are there. I guess it's pretty well just up to me. George will do what he can, but he's not able to do everything."

"OK, Mr. Marshall. Let's see what we've got. You're going to be a bit weak for a while, and you're going to need some assistance until you get your strength back. I've read your medical records and, as you've been told, your prognosis is very good, so you can expect to get better. Mr. Clark says that he thinks you are a pretty tough, independent person."

"Ordinarily, I do pretty well, Miz . . . Carroll, didn't you say your name was?" Mr. Marshall is obviously pleased with the supportive evaluation of his personality.

"Right. Carroll. You're going to hear it a lot for a while," says Ms. Carroll with another smile.

"Mr. Marshall, I'm going to need you to help me with a couple of things. I'd like to visit your house to see how it is laid out. Stairs, kitchen, and bathroom mostly. Would you be willing to ask George to meet me there some evening after he gets off work?"

"Sure, I guess so."

"OK then, let me take a look. Once I get an idea of how things are, I'll talk to you about what we can do to help you recover. There are a number of services we can use, and next time I'll tell you about them. I come to the hospital regularly, so I'll see you in a few days."

"I'll be here, I guess. And I'm sorry I was surprised. I didn't mean to . . ."

"It's all right, Mr. Marshall. I think we can work together, don't you?"

"Yes. Sure. You're a nice lady."

"Well, let's see how I do before you make up your mind, Mr. Marshall. I'm going to leave now, since I hear them banging the lunch trays. I want to get out of here before I have to look at the food," says Ms. Carroll, laughing.

"At least you don't have to eat it," Mr. Marshall responds, laughing with her.

Ms. Carroll met George at Mr. Marshall's small house the next night. She found that the house was all on one floor with the bathroom located conveniently across the hall from Mr. Marshall's bedroom. A second, small bedroom was tucked next to the bathroom. There was no dining room, but there was a dining alcove in one end of the kitchen. This opened into a small but neatly furnished living room. The kitchen did not have all the appliances that one might want, but there was a refrigerator with a small freezer in the top, an electric stove with an oven, a toaster, and a blender. While the appliances were not new, all were in good working order.

George Marshall was a quiet, middle-aged man. The family resemblance was slight. Where Mr. Marshall was tall and thin, George was short and stout.

"Well, what do you think, Ms. Carroll?" asked George Marshall after he had shown her the house.

"I think it will do just fine, Mr. Marshall. Your father won't be able to do very much for a while, but he'll get stronger as time goes on. He's a pretty tough old bird, anyway."

"Yeah. Those skinny guys will fool you. Pop always was a hard worker."

"Realistically, Mr. Marshall, will you be able to be of help to your father?" asked Ms. Carroll.

"Well, I can't be here all the time. I'm a foreman at the candy works—the Sally Jane plant."

"Don't take offense, Mr. Marshall, but I do have to know just how much time you can give to your father's care."

"No offense taken," said George, "I understand that you are trying to figure out what I can and can't do so you'll know what has to be filled in, right?"

"Right."

"Well, I can come over most evenings and maybe fix a meal and help him get ready for bed. I may not be able to do it every night, though, since I do sometimes work overtime. And I do have a social life of sorts. I'm pretty much a loner, but I bowl on Tuesdays."

"Does Mr. Marshall have any close friends nearby?"

"Well, yes, sort of."

"Do you want to tell me about it, or am I pushing too hard?" said Ms. Carroll.

"Oh, no. It's kind of silly, I suppose, but Dad has kind of a relationship with Millie Pearce down the block."

"And you don't approve?"

"Oh, it's not that. It's just that—at Dad's age, isn't it a little, well, pointless? I mean, what are they going to do with each other?"

"Love each other, maybe, Mr. Marshall. Or just like each other some. It's not unheard of."

"Yeah. Well. Anyway, there it is."

"As you say, Mr. Marshall, there it is," said Ms. Carroll as she turned to leave. "Good night, Mr. Marshall. Thank you for taking the time."

"Good night, Ms. Carroll. I hope we can get Dad squared away."

"We will, Mr. Marshall. I'll call you soon. I've got a couple of other things to look into, but I think it will work out."

Two days later, Ms. Carroll was at the hospital. She stopped in to see Mr. Marshall, who was sitting up in a chair drinking a glass of orange juice.

"Best thing they fix here," he said, finishing the glass.

"That's probably right," said Ms. Carroll.

"Well, what's going to become of me?" asked Mr. Marshall, his hand shaking slightly as he put down the glass.

"Are you worried about something?" Ms. Carroll's Canadian "aboot" seemed to tickle Mr. Marshall despite his agitation.

"I'm worried 'aboot' being put in a nursing home," he said with a nervous laugh.

"I see that I need to talk to you about nursing homes sometime, Mr. Marshall. I think you've been reading the wrong stuff."

"Well, I can't help but wonder. I know I'm not well yet and I still hurt like hell sometimes."

"Surgery hurts, I don't care what they say, Mr. Marshall."

"So what are you going to do?"

"*I'm* not going to do anything. *We're* going to talk about your options," said Ms. Carroll with her customary warm smile.

"What choice have I got?" Mr. Marshall showed bitterness for the first time.

"Mainly two, Mr. Marshall. First, the hospital would like to discharge you on Monday."

"That's pretty soon, isn't it?" said Mr. Marshall, looking a bit frightened.

"About average, Mr. Marshall. You've actually progressed very well."

"But I'm still weak as a cat."

"You feel weak, I expect, but you are mending. And you'll probably improve faster after you leave."

"Am I one of those getting out quicker and sicker?"

"Mr. Marshall, it's true that modern medical practice does send people home much sooner than used to be the case. In a sense, yes, they are sicker. On the other hand, what usually happens is that the patient repairs quicker at home."

"So they are going to send me home. How will I manage?"

"Whoa, Mr. Marshall. Home is one option."

"And the other?"

"Skilled nursing care for a couple of weeks, and then home."

"In a nursing home?"

"In a very good nursing home where I will be keeping track of your care on a regular basis. That's my job."

"I don't like the idea of a nursing home."

"Nursing home, Mr. Marshall, not snake pit. I wouldn't refer you to a place that wasn't all right. That's my job, too," smiled Ms. Carroll. The Jamaican lilt was coming back into her voice.

"Well, if I went home, how would I manage?"

"First, my agency will provide home health care. This includes regular visits from a registered nurse and a home health aide. The nurse will check on your health, and the aide will help you bathe and shave.

"Second, a homemaker from Family Service will come by once a week and clean up, change the sheets, and do the laundry.

"Third, you'll get a hot meal delivered at noon and the same person will leave you a sandwich and some soup George can warm for supper. George will come over most nights—except Tuesday—and keep you company for a while. How does it sound so far?"

"Expensive. How can I afford it?"

"Medicare for the home health care, a small fee for the homemaker service, and a contribution for the hot meal if you are willing to pay something. George is free." (I'm smiling a lot, thought Ms. Carroll. My face is beginning to hurt!)

"Actually, that doesn't sound so bad," said Mr. Marshall looking more relaxed than he had.

"One more thing. I talked to Mrs. Millie Pearce. Seems she wants to look in on you from time to time."

"You talked to Millie?"

"Sure. George said it was all right. Besides, she's been in to visit you here, hasn't she? Nurse on the floor says she's a pretty nice lady."

"Oh, yes, it's all right. I just didn't think that she'd want to be burdened. She had to do so much for her husband before he died that I figured that she had enough of sick old men."

"Don't think she looks at it that way. Seems to think you're an entertaining fellow. She says she enjoys your company."

"Well, I'll be damned. Maybe it will work out."

"It's supposed to."

"But what if it doesn't?"

"I'll be by once a week to see that it does."

"For how long?"

"Until you're safely back on your feet."

"You're a pretty tough cookie, yourself, aren't you Miz Carroll?"

"Bet your boots, Mr. Marshall. You get some sleep now. I got a really tough case to visit, and I need to get going."

In this illustration, we have included the relevant elements of the case manager's role. Ms. Carroll used her knowledge of Mr. Marshall's health and social situation to develop alternatives for him to consider. It is, after all, his choice. Included in her assessment of the situation was a visit with George Marshall and a visit to Mr. Marshall's home in order to assess the feasibility of a return to it. Had the home been in poor repair with dangerous stairways and ill-functioning appliances, going home would have been a much less attractive option.

Because of Mr. Marshall's small family system, Ms. Carroll properly looked for friends that could be of help. If Mrs. Pearce had a previous relationship with Mr. Marshall, she probably would have looked in on him anyway, but as a case manager, Ms. Carroll needed to know of her interest and take it into account as part of the social support available to Mr. Marshall. She also explored George's ability to help, but didn't try to make him feel guilty and didn't ask him to do more than he was willing to do.

In her professional role as a case manager, Ms. Carroll developed a plan (two plans, actually) that included the services of a number of agencies. Part of her service will include helping Mr. Marshall fill out any applications required. She will assist in filling out any insurance papers that need to be submitted as well. If he needs transportation for follow-up medical visits, Ms. Carroll will arrange it as well.

When Mr. Marshall goes home, Ms. Carroll will see to it that the plan is carried out. If there are problems, Mr. Marshall will call Ms. Carroll. He will not have to run down the "bugs" in the system himself, but can devote his time to getting well. She will monitor his progress and is prepared to suggest changes in the mix of services when that is appropriate.

Ms. Carroll also had to deal with a bit of racism in the client. We didn't make it serious, but we did want to create the opportunity to raise the question. Unfortunately, professionals of ethnic and racial groups different from that of the client or patient may still experience varying degrees of bias or resistance. They must deal with these problems on an everyday basis. In this case, Ms. Carroll was able to minimize the problem easily. Had she not been able to do this or had Mr. Marshall been more difficult about the matter, it might have been necessary to transfer the service to another professional. This should only be done as a last resort, in our view. We think that it is far better for both patient and service provider to work it out unless the situation is clearly harmful for one or the other of them. The relationships between ethnic and racial groups will never be totally resolved unless we face them in the context of everyday life and learn to accept each other as fellow human beings with legitimate roles to fill.

As we mentioned earlier, the case management system is probably not always as good as it ought to be. Our Ms. Carroll is unusually good at her job, and we think that she represents what good case management should be.

Human Services in the Long-Term Care Facility

An estimated 5 percent of elderly persons live in long-term care facilities. These people are usually seriously ill or disabled and require care that would be difficult or impossible outside of a specialized facility.

Contrary to popular opinion, Americans do not "dump" their older family members in nursing homes. Nursing home care is sought when other alternatives have been exhausted. This is unfortunate, since a good nursing home can be a reasonable option and not just a last resort. Generally, most people take the position that one should try to avoid institutional care if at all possible. Support groups, respite care services, and the kinds of community-based systems that Ms. Carroll suggested to Mr. Marshall allow many people to remain in their own homes, which most Americans still prefer.

In some cases, the older person will request nursing home care because he or she "does not want to be a burden." This motivation is not healthy, in our view, since it is suggestive of some disorder in the family system. In other cases, some older persons believe, rightly at times, that they will have more independence in a nursing home than they will have if they live with relatives. This, too, has unhealthy overtones, since it suggests that the older person's role in the family is not terribly secure.

The choice of whether to use a nursing home or to maintain the older person in his or her own home is a difficult one. Part of the problem is the general suspicion of nursing homes. (Recall Mr. Marshall's apprehension in our example.)

In order to discuss the nursing home as a resource for the frail older person, some distinctions need to be made between nursing homes and those institutions that are not nursing homes but are often confused with them.

There are institutions in many places that are called boarding homes or rest homes. Often, these places are converted old houses that offer care for anywhere from four or five people up to a dozen or more, depending on the number of beds that can be accommodated. Unfortunately, in many states, these boarding homes are not subject to the same licensing laws that regulate true nursing homes. We have seen some that are decently run, but in far too many the standards of care are shockingly low. Of course, they charge less for care, and this is their sole attractiveness.

Some of the residents really need a higher level of care than that provided, but either their relatives cannot or will not provide it. Sadly, some of these people may be eligible for Medicaid, but either do not know it or they have caretakers who are unwilling to apply for it.

Some of these boarding homes do, in fact, become dumping grounds for unwanted or unliked elders. More likely, they are used because of their cost.

A nursing home, on the other hand, must meet state standards that specify a certain level of care. Staff must have some level of professional qualification and the institution must provide a decent diet, clean facilities, and be able to ensure the safety of the occupants. In addition, most reputable nursing homes belong to the American Health Care Association, which has standards for membership. Further, if the nursing home is to receive Medicare or Medicaid payments, it must qualify by meeting federal standards. The latter requirement has resulted in relatively uniform national standards. Consequently, one should be able to expect a certain level of humane care from a licensed nursing home that accepts Medicare and Medicaid patients. There are many other good nursing homes that provide high-quality care, but only accept patients or residents that can afford to pay private rates. We will have some hints on selecting a nursing home later in this chapter, but first we want to illustrate how a good nursing home operates and the role of the service professional in the long-term care institution.

The Nursing Home as a Resource

We believe that the nursing home should be regarded as a specialized resource that is part of the array of services available to older persons. The nursing home should be used as the facility of choice when the individual needs a higher amount of specialized care than can be provided at home. Generally, there are two levels of care. Usually, both levels are offered in the same facility, but this is not necessarily so. Intermediate care denotes a level of care in which the individual needs considerable assistance with the activities of daily living and consistent but not constant attention. Skilled care, on the other hand, indicates a level of care that is much more intensive because of serious medical problems.

We will show you how we think a good nursing home should operate by accompanying Charles and Mary Davis as they discuss the feasibility of admission of Mr. Davis' aunt, Mrs. Marjorie Parker.

Mrs. Parker is eighty-five. She has lived alone in the house that she and her late husband bought in 1931. The Parkers had two children. Elaine, age fifty-six, is the older. She and her husband have recently retired and are living in a small town in the Florida panhandle, near

Fort Walton Beach. Elaine is concerned about her mother, but is too far away to help effectively. Jeff, age sixty-one, lives in town, and he and his wife find themselves with the major burden of deciding about care for Mrs. Parker. The trouble is that Mrs. Parker's arthritic condition has steadily worsened, and she can no longer manage to live independently. The solutions that worked for Mr. Marshall do not appear to be appropriate, since Mrs. Parker simply needs more assistance than he did and her condition is likely to become worse with time. Accordingly, Jeff has asked his cousin Charles to help by visiting several nursing homes. Jeff figures that Charles, being a nephew, can be a bit more objective. Besides, Charles is cynical and hard to please, and Jeff believes that he will ask the right questions about how Mrs. Parker will be treated.

Mr. and Mrs. Davis enter a small but neat office where they are greeted by Ms. Chavez, the staff social worker. Ms. Chavez is a calm young woman who is neatly dressed in a rust-colored shirtwaist dress. She wears no white coat or nameplate, preferring to avoid the "institutional look." Since they have come by appointment, Ms. Chavez has had some advance notice of their situation and has, with Mrs. Parker's consent, obtained the family physician's evaluation of her condition.

After introducing herself, Ms. Chavez says, "Please sit down, Mr. and Mrs. Davis. I understand you're inquiring about Hillsdale on behalf of your aunt. Would you like me to explain our services, or would you prefer to ask questions?"

"Well, we do have a lot of questions, but I'm afraid that they are not in good order. We're looking at several nursing homes, but Hillsdale is the first on the list."

"You are wise to visit a number of nursing homes, Mr. Davis. It is not an easy decision, I know, so it should be made carefully. I gather that the family has discussed this at some length."

"Yes," says Mrs. Davis, "Aunt Marjorie realizes that she is unable to manage at home. It's probably most accurate to say that she has reluctantly concluded that she needs more care than the family can give her, even with the help of home health care services."

"Most of us have trouble accepting the limits that time imposes on us, so that is quite understandable," says Ms. Chavez softly.

"I guess that it is something that most of us will face sometime," says Mr. Davis.

"Maybe it will help if I give you a brief description of what we have here and then I'll show you around the facility. Please ask any questions, and I'll try to answer them," says Ms. Chavez.

The Davises nod their agreement.

"First, there are some general things that you need to know. We are licensed by the state, and are members of the American Health Care Association. We are also approved for Medicare and Medicaid reimbursement. What all this means is that we meet state and federal standards for the quality of our care, and that we are associated with a national organization. The practical meaning is that we are regularly inspected."

"But don't all nursing homes have to be inspected?" asks Mrs. Davis.

"Yes, if they operate as nursing homes and take federal reimbursements."

"Aunt Marjorie has Medicare, of course, but will it cover her care here?"

"No, Mr. Davis. Although she will need assistance in living, she does not need skilled care."

"Then she and the family will be responsible for the cost?"

"Yes, Mr. Davis, they will."

"Well, I don't want to appear crass, Ms. Chavez, but I guess we'll have to know about the cost before we go any further."

"Certainly. Cost is a factor, and it's quite understandable that you need to ask about it. Our basic charge for intermediate care is $1,685 per month. This includes nursing care, a semi-private room, meals, and laundry."

The Davises look thoughtful. Ms. Chavez waits for their questions and does not press them for their response.

"Just hearing the figure, it seems like a lot of money," says Mr. Davis.

"Yes, it is," says Ms. Chavez.

"All right, so what exactly would the Parkers get for the money?" says Mr. Davis.

"First of all, Mrs. Parker will get a semi-private room with a bath that she will share with another woman. We try to bring compatible people together as roommates, but just as is the case with college roommates or bunkmates in the service, it doesn't always work out, and we try to respond to requests for changes. She will have assistance in bathing and toileting if that is necessary. Since she is able to walk some days and can use a wheelchair, she will be encouraged to eat in our dining room. On days when she can't manage, we'll bring her a tray, but we encourage our residents to get up and around as much as possible. We encourage them to get dressed every day unless they are acutely ill. Our head nurse believes that residents do better when they get up and around."

"But what if they don't want to? Suppose someone just wants to mooch around in a bathrobe all day?" asks Mrs. Davis.

"Ms. Benedict, our head nurse, gives in gracefully on occasion, but she is pretty firm in her belief that it is generally not healthy to take to your bed and not get out. To be candid, I think you should know as much as you can about the staff's general philosophy of care as you visit nursing homes."

"While we're at it, how do you come into the picture? I thought social workers worked with the poor," says Mr. Davis.

"Some of us do. Most of us have specialties nowadays, and our education varies. My specialization is working with older people and their families. Here I do a variety of things. First, I do a lot of what I'm doing now—explain the services the nursing home offers to prospective residents and their families. I also take social histories of incoming residents. Basically, a social history is a description of who the resident is as a human being. It helps the staff to know the resident better so that we can, as best we are able, tailor our care to him or her.

"I also spend a lot of time talking to the residents. I try to help them talk about their concerns, and I try to help them deal with their problems in living here and in their relationships with their families.

"I also talk to families of residents. They need to know how the resident is getting along and how they can best be supportive. Sometimes, this involves referring family members to various sources of information and help."

"So you would be available to discuss things with the Parkers if any problems were to arise?"

"Yes."

"And are there usually problems?"

"Yes, frankly. I would not give you false assurance. We have 140 beds. This requires a big staff—about seventy nurses alone—working three shifts. Any time you have that many people in close proximity every day, you will have problems."

"I guess we've never thought about that, Ms. Chavez," says Mrs. Davis.

"I don't mean to emphasize the problems, Mrs. Davis, but you do need to know that people in a nursing home are still people and they bring with them a lifetime of habits, beliefs, and values. People go on being what they were. And although the staff are professionals, they are not immune from being affected by turf problems and personal likes and dislikes."

"Just one big, happy family, eh?" says Mr. Davis with a smile.

"I'm afraid so," says Ms. Chavez, smiling with him. "Becoming old and ill does not rescue us from being what we are."

"Are many of the patients, well, you know, senile?" asks Mrs. Davis.

"Yes, Mrs. Davis, some patients do suffer from what the doctors call dementias—Alzheimer's disease, for example. Most of them are in the wing reserved for skilled care, because they require a great deal of help. There are a few mild cases in the sections for intermediate care, but they will, as you probably know, get worse."

"That brings up the question of medical care. How is that handled?" asks Mr. Davis.

"All of our residents are admitted following a physician's referral. We expect that they will continue to be seen regularly by their physicians, although we do have internists that we call in emergencies. Some nursing homes have a staff physician, but we do not. We would rather work with the resident's regular doctor. Of course, if the resident wants to change doctors, we'll work with whomever they choose."

"How about visiting?"

"We encourage visitors. We suggest that visitors come during the afternoon and early evening, since, frankly, it makes it easier for the staff to clean, change beds, and do the routine care. However, there's no hard and fast rule about it, and if it is more convenient for the family and friends, they can come any time. They might have to put up with some clutter, of course."

"Will Aunt Marjorie be able to leave?"

"Oh, yes," Ms. Chavez smiles. "She can come and go as she likes as long as she is able. Since she does have trouble getting around we will ask that she leave with some responsible person. We just can't let residents go off on their own; I'm sure you can understand that."

"Actually, I don't think we in the family would want you to turn her out of doors without company!" laughs Mr. Davis.

"Aunt Marjorie likes to go shopping at the mall when she's feeling good," says Mrs. Davis.

"No reason she can't continue to do it," says Ms. Chavez.

"How about going out at night—say to a play or something?"

"Nothing to stop that either. In fact, sometimes we borrow the bus from St. Michael's, now that Father John has found someone to repair it, and take as many residents as we can to things. We can't take everybody, of course, since there is only one bus and St. Michael's uses it a lot, but we try to take people who are able to things that interest them when we can. Mostly, we depend on the resident's family to provide the outside recreation, though, since we use our resources primarily for patient care."

"Do you have a recreational program in the home?" asks Mr. Davis.

"Yes, we do, Mr. Davis. But it may not be what you might expect," answers Ms. Chavez.

"What do you mean?"

"First, for those residents who are willing and able, we provide the opportunity for exercise. While we don't have a bus, we do have a physical therapist. Besides carrying out doctor's orders for specific exercise, he offers group sessions tailored to the residents' activity level. We also do a lot of walking in the neighborhood. If your aunt comes to live here, we'll suggest that you take her for walks when she feels up to it. At least, go for a walk in our rose garden when the roses are in bloom.

"Second, we encourage the residents to continue those things they considered recreation before they came here. We have, for example, a regular duplicate bridge group that is sanctioned by the American Contract Bridge Association, so the points count."

"I don't know what that means," says Mrs. Davis.

"Bridge players do, though, dear," says Mr. Davis who has never succeeded in persuading his wife to play.

"We have room for people who want to sew, paint, play musical instruments—pretty much whatever they have been accustomed to doing. We don't make anybody do anything, however, and we do not promote amateur theatricals nor do we have a kazoo band."

"I've seen some of that on television," says Mrs. Davis, "and it always seems cute and contrived."

"The staff shares your view, Mrs. Davis. After talking it over, we decided that our policy would be to try to make it possible for the residents to do what they wanted to do instead of what we thought they ought to do. Sometimes, that's simply reading, watching TV, or sitting near the front door to see who's coming in or going out."

"Let's take a look around, now, Ms. Chavez, if you don't mind, so we can report back to Jeff."

"Certainly," says Ms. Chavez.

Ms. Chavez' office is to the left of the entrance hall. Hillsdale Center is a one-story building that resembles a large capital *E* with greatly elongated legs. The building sits in a wooded area on the edge of town, about a mile from the mall, the largest shopping center in the community. The long side of the building faces the highway, but is about 200 yards back from the building setback line. The legs of the *E* contain the residents' rooms. Two legs are for intermediate care, and the third contains the rooms for skilled care. A separate building contains the furnace and air-conditioning equipment and a repair shop.

Ms. Chavez turns left in the long corridor that connects the residents' wings. To the right is the kitchen. An enormous glass window allows one to see the kitchen staff preparing the evening meal. A tall man in a chef's hat is gesturing with a beef fork while two assistants slice onions and carrots. Two women are preparing salads on a stainless steel table.

The dining room is furnished with small tables that each seat four people. The wall facing the inside courtyard between wings one and two is thermopane with drapes that can be opened and closed. The view is of a small rock garden with trees in pots, a paved walk with benches, and an occasional lamppost. The area is only about fifty feet across, but gives the impression of spaciousness because of the curved walk. Several older people can be seen walking and sitting on the benches.

The dining room itself is painted a neutral beige, but bright hangings and paintings are on the walls. The room is brightly lit with lights flush-mounted into the ceiling tile. The tables have cloths in several colors—bright reds, greens, blues, and oranges. The tables are not geometrically arranged, but have a certain pleasing irregularity. All chairs have high backs and each has sturdy arms. Several large pots containing healthy, large green plants have been placed in the corners of the room.

"Very pleasant," says Mrs. Davis.

They turn into a long corridor at the end of the dining room. On the right, there is a small lounge furnished as a living room in a private home. Newspapers and magazines are strewn about. Although the room is clean, it has a cluttered look. Two men are bent over a checkerboard. They look up and wave to Ms. Chavez and smile at the visitors, then turn back to their game.

"This lounge is used primarily for socializing," says Ms. Chavez softly, "although Mr. Carrillo and Mr. Weller don't look very sociable right now. I think they're playing a grudge match! There is a similar lounge in each wing."

"And you don't apologize for the clutter, thank God," says Mr. Davis.

"These rooms get cluttered, Mr. Davis. We keep them clean, but frankly, we don't try to keep them looking like showrooms. We try to operate on the philosophy that people live here."

To the left is a small chapel. It is simply furnished with pine pews. In the front is a small table covered with a green cloth that reaches the floor on all sides. On the table is an open Bible flanked by a bare cross, a crucifix, and a Star of David. Bouquets of fresh flowers rest on small stands at each side of the table.

Ms. Chavez explains, "Several local clergymen take turns conducting services for Protestant residents here at 10:30 on Sunday. A rabbi comes in on Friday evening for services. For Catholic residents, one of the young priests from the cathedral says Mass at 8:00 on Sunday mornings. Of course, some residents are able to attend services at their regular places of worship, but most use the chapel.

"Some of our residents come here just to sit quietly or pray. We have two atheists who come in here regularly just because it is a quiet place to think. We have a lot of deaths here, you understand. Often families arrange for funerals to be held here. Even when they don't, we hold a brief service of remembrance for each resident who dies. Some nursing homes like to pretend that no one dies. We think that is unrealistic. Residents often know when someone has died before most of the staff do. We don't discourage residents from grieving for friends they have lost."

As they proceed down the corridor, rooms with closed doors can be seen on each side. There are two nurses' stations at intervals down the hall. A glassed-in sunroom is visible at the far end of the hall, and the sound of chatter drifts down the hall. Although the corridor is long, there are skylights at intervals, relieving the closed-in feeling that one might get otherwise.

"I'm going to show you a vacant room. We don't like to intrude on our residents' privacy. A closed door tells us to stay out unless it's meal time or there is a need to talk to the resident."

As they speak, a uniformed nurse approaches them, smiles, and then taps at a closed door.

"Miss Jamieson? May I come in?" says the nurse.

"Yes, come in, please," says a gravelly voice from within the room.

The nurse opens the door and goes into the room, closing it behind him.

"Is everyone trained by Miss Manners here?" asks Mrs. Davis.

Ms. Chavez laughs. "Well, yes, we do try to stress courtesy. We try to treat each resident with respect, although tempers do get short on occasion. We've found that it is healthier for both residents and staff, so yes, most of the time we make a conscious effort to be a bit formal, particularly about the privacy of the resident."

"I notice that nobody is on a first-name basis. Is that part of it?"

"Yes, it is. When I worked in a hospital in Illinois, the staff called most of the older people by their first names. It was as if they were small children. When I came here for a job interview, I was impressed with the effect of being more respectful of the older person. It's simply more professional to be courteous. Older people are not small children. In our case, they are also customers, in a way, and they can move if they do not feel well treated."

Ms. Chavez opens the door to a clean, airy room with two beds, two dressing tables, and two closets. There are two sets of drawers built into the wall across from each bed. At the far end of the room there is a small love seat, a coffee table, and two comfortable chairs.

"Very large room," comments Mr. Davis.

"We also have some private rooms, but they are smaller, and we charge a bit more for them," says Ms. Chavez.

"Is there a difference between the rooms for people who pay their own way and those who are on Medicaid?"

"No. About one-third of our residents are on Medicaid. Some nursing homes have a higher proportion of Medicaid-supported residents. I'll be very honest with you about this. Our private-pay residents' fees do reflect some subsidy of the Medicaid residents. Our fees would actually be lower if we didn't accept Medicaid patients, but we believe we should do what we can to serve the whole community. The nursing home is a business, Mr. Davis, but we are not without a sense of obligation to human need. Fortunately, we also have a growing endowment fund that provides income to assist some residents who otherwise could not afford to stay here."

After they have looked at the room, Ms. Chavez takes them back to the main wing and shows them several rooms in which people are engaged in various activities. In one, two women are painting pictures of a bowl of fruit set on a table draped with black cloth. A young man is looking on, and he comments from time to time.

"He's a volunteer from the university. Art student who comes by on Thursdays."

A door leads into a small hallway with several small rooms that open off it. The Davises can faintly hear a badly played saxophone.

"Practice rooms," Ms. Chavez explains, "and soundproofed for our musical residents, thank heavens!"

Another room is an awful clutter of tables with all manner of junk strewn about. One table has an electric fan that has been disassembled. A tall, thin man is peering at the motor and muttering under his breath. Another bench contains a lawnmower engine in pieces and a greasy array of tools. Others have unidentifiable objects in various stages of completion. At one, an older woman dressed in coveralls is assembling a bird feeder from a kit. Standing next to her and looking on is a university student. Two leathery-looking older men seated on high stools at one workbench are patiently sanding the persimmon heads of some ancient wooden golf clubs. Everybody in the room seems to be talking at once.

"Is everybody expected to do something here?" asks Mr. Davis.

"No. We have our share of couch potatoes! And quite a few of our patients are too ill to be interested in much activity. But we do have people who like to putter, so we try to provide them with a place to do it. We don't have a TV lounge or a large day room as some nursing homes do. We've just used the space differently," says Ms. Chavez as she leads them back to the office.

"Well, thank you very much for your time, Ms. Chavez. We'll report on what we've seen to Jeff and Aunt Marjorie."

"Here is our brochure, Mr. Davis. It describes Hillsdale and it may be useful. If Hillsdale seems right for your aunt, I hope you'll bring her for a visit before the family makes its decision. Thank you for coming."

Discussion

We have again "seeded" this fictional example with several points that we want to emphasize. You will note that we have created an idealized situation. Most good nursing homes will have some of the features that we have incorporated into Hillsdale, but few will have all of them. Even the good ones cannot conceal their institutional aspects, and persons who work in them or who refer potential residents to them will find that most nursing homes will have their share of ill-tempered patients, disenchanted staff members, and bureaucratic administrators engaged in infighting over privilege and power. In short, nursing homes are not much different from other organizations.

In spite of that, most nursing homes do provide good care to persons who need it. One should not automatically equate them with the more bizarre models portrayed on television or in horror stories.

Ms. Chavez gave the Davises good advice when she agreed that they should visit a number of nursing homes. She also suggested that Mrs. Parker make some visits as they identified the nursing homes that looked good to them. This practice works well if there is no great hurry to find a nursing home placement. Unfortunately, as mentioned earlier, many families choose nursing homes at a time of crisis and do not have the luxury of comparison shopping. In some communities nursing home beds are in short supply, and families may be forced (at least initially) to take whatever is available.

Money, too, is a problem. Most nursing homes will, if they are qualified, have a sizable proportion of long-term residents whose care is paid by Medicaid. Most do as Hillsdale does—subsidize the Medicaid patients with the fees charged to non-Medicaid patients. Medicaid does not pay enough to provide the quality of care that Hillsdale—and many of its real-life counterparts—provides.

The Davises also learned something about the role of the social service professional on their visit. Most large nursing homes have some provision for full-time social service staff. Smaller homes may hire a social worker on a part-time basis or will at least have a consultant who can assist other staff in accomplishing some of the tasks that Ms. Chavez performs.

Ms. Chavez said a lot about the staff's general philosophy of patient care. As a general rule, the nursing home staff will try to get patients up and dressed and will not let them stay in bed unless they are acutely ill. They will try to encourage the residents to go to the dining room for meals. Many nursing homes will not have the elaborate and permissive recreational opportunities that Hillsdale has, but our idealism prompted us to add those amenities. We wish that nursing homes did have the room to allow ambulatory patients more self-selected activity. We know of some that offer the patient a great deal of freedom to putter, but most just don't have the space. Others do provide more organized activity, but sometimes this degenerates into busy work that is of no meaningful purpose to the residents.

We have emphasized our conviction that older persons should be treated with respect and dignity, and should be allowed privacy even in institutions that must medically supervise their activity. Sick people do not stop being people, and they should not be demeaned because they are ill. They should not be forced into activity they do not like. Of course, attractive activity should be available and gently encouraged for health reasons, but it should have meaning for the participants.

Most good nursing homes work with the residents' regular physicians. Physicians make regular rounds and respond to patient needs. These nursing homes take the patient to the doctor when routine care is needed and the patient is able to go.

We decorated Hillsdale with bright colors and let in lots of natural light. This is consistent with our discussion in chapter 6. We also tolerated considerable clutter. Some real nursing homes are too antiseptic. Residents may be afraid to use facilities that are too neat. We think that it is possible to keep an institution fundamentally clean, yet informal enough for residents to be able to use it.

Hillsdale has a brochure. Some nursing homes do and others do not, but all will have some kind of description of their services and how much they cost. Persons selecting a nursing home and professionals who refer people to them need to know what types of patients the home accepts, what services are available, and their cost in order to make rational decisions.

Choosing a Nursing Home

As a professional in aging, you are likely to be asked about nursing homes by older people and their families. There are some simple things that can be easily ascertained that will help separate the good from the poor choices. We have hinted at most of these in the preceding discussion, but some are mentioned here for the first time.

1. Consider only those nursing homes that are licensed. As we said earlier, licensing laws vary, but they do offer some minimal assurance of quality of staff and level of care. Medicare and Medicaid eligibility are another indication of basic quality, but again we stress that some good nursing homes choose not to accept Medicaid or Medicare patients, so this is not a universal guide. Membership in the American Health Care Association is also an indication of the institution's concern with quality.

None of the above factors is an absolute indicator of quality, so there are other things that one can look at.

2. Smell the air! A well-run nursing home does not have an offensive odor. Of course, there will be incontinent patients, and patients with various odor-producing conditions. However, an institution with a good staff will keep the patients clean, the sheets changed, and the laundry done to the point where there will be little or no noticeable smell. Smell, prosaic as it may sound, is a good indicator of quality of care. A persistently bad-smelling nursing home has too few staff or bad staff morale. Therefore, it is badly run.

3. Examine the fee schedule carefully. Make sure that you know what services are included and what are not. Beware of hidden charges.

4. Ask to see the kitchen. A good nursing home will let you see anything. A nursing home operator that restricts potential residents and their families to the office or a few public rooms may have something to hide.

5. Talk to the staff and try to observe them in action. It is particularly important to have contact with the aides, since it is they, not the R.N., the administrator, or the social worker, who spend the most time in direct contact with the residents. The way they treat the current patients is the way they will treat the person on whose behalf you are inquiring.

6. Find out what will happen if the resident's regular doctor is unavailable. A good nursing home will have a satisfactory back-up plan for emergencies.

7. Observe the residents. Given that most of them may have chronic, painful conditions and may not be the most cheerful humans as a consequence, they still should show signs of good—or poor—care.

8. Find out about visiting hours and any restrictions on activity. A good nursing home will accommodate itself to residents who wish to come and go and to family schedules, unless the demands are unreasonable.

9. Ask about choices. A good nursing home will encourage residents to make choices about activities, preferences for foods, and furnishings in the resident's room. Within reason, they will allow the resident to bring treasured objects from home.

10. Finally, ask others about the nursing home. Find people whose relatives are or have been residents recently or ask a physician whose judgment can be trusted in such matters.

In addition to the above points, one will still have to think about the home's location and the fundamental compatibility of the residents with the staff and the environment.

A good nursing home is a valuable resource for persons who need what it has to offer. Approach the choice with the potential resident's needs and wants clearly in mind.

Postscript

By the time you read this postscript, we expect that you will be near completion of a course designed to help prepare you for work with older persons and their families. We hope that you are seriously considering a career in aging. The need for highly motivated, well-prepared persons to work in the field of aging is great. This course, together with others you will take, as well as an experience in which you actually come in contact with older persons and their families should provide a good beginning to guide your learning about how best to help people age successfully.

But your formal education should be only a beginning. Over the years, we have been amazed at the development of knowledge about the processes of aging and at the development of policies and programs to help people age successfully. We fully expect continuing development of knowledge, policies, and programs in the years ahead.

This is why it is vitally important that anyone intending to make a career of working with older persons make a commitment to staying well informed about advances in gerontology and strategies for helping people age successfully. There are several ways to do this, and we encourage you to make use of all of them.

Keep Up with the Professional Literature

Make professional reading related to your job a regular part of your life. In virtually all professional fields that deal with older persons, there is now at least one journal that deals specifically with work with the elderly. We urge you to subscribe to that journal or to make arrangements to read it regularly at your agency or a local library. This is an excellent way to keep up to date with what is current in gerontology as it relates to your specific profession. Also, we commend highly to you *The Gerontologist*, a bimonthly publication of the Gerontological Society of America. This journal includes research articles, discussions of practice, book reviews, and reviews of audiovisual materials likely to be of interest to anyone making a career in gerontology. The book review sections of this and other journals on aging provide an excellent way for you to decide which books you want to add to your own or your agency's professional library. You should also try to get on the mailing list of the National Institute on Aging. This federally sponsored agency periodically distributes information about the latest research on aging. This information can be of help to you and to the people with whom you work.

With the demands of day-to-day activities, it is sometimes difficult to add professional reading to everything else that must be done. In some agencies, the importance of professional reading is highlighted by having staff members give brief reviews of what they have read recently at regular staff meetings. In others, a special monthly lunch is held at which there is discussion of the implications of one article that all attendees have read.

Become Active in Gerontological Societies

Many states have organized gerontological societies, membership groups of professionals and others interested in older persons. These societies sponsor annual meetings and other conferences and professional meetings. Attending these provides you with the opportunity to meet with others in the field of aging, to listen to them talk about service innovations developed in their communities, and generally to share information that will help you become a better, more knowledgeable professional. The Gerontological Society of America and the American Society on Aging are two national organizations that have annual conferences, bringing together professionals in aging from throughout the nation. Each annual meeting affords an excellent opportunity for you to learn what is new all over the country.

Attend Continuing Education Programs

Many agencies, colleges, and universities offer continuing education programs in aging. Sometimes these are highly focused (for example, working with spouses of Alzheimer's disease patients) and can help you as you take on new responsibilities within your agency. It is common for agencies to assist with the costs of travel and registration to attend continuing education programs, particularly when the agencies do not themselves offer specialized training. As you learn of these opportunities, discuss them with your supervisor and try to make arrangements to attend those related to what you do.

Develop Good Contacts with Other Professionals in Your Community

There is no substitute for being knowledgeable about the agencies and services available in the community where you work. To stay knowledgeable, it is important to be in touch with others who provide services to older persons in your community. Usually, there are regular meetings of groups of professionals in a community that facilitate this kind of informal contact. In one city that we know of, professionals from all fields interested in the aging meet monthly for lunch. One member describes his or her agency's services, with a special focus on innovations and changes in policies. Those attending the lunch benefit not only from the formal program, but also from the informal contacts they make just by getting together.

We urge you, as you get involved in your career, to remember that your education is by no means over when you receive your diploma. It has just begun. While personal experience is a demanding teacher, much is to be gained by learning from others through the published literature and through contacts with others who are struggling, as you are, with the same issues, problems, and joys of helping people age successfully.

References

American Association of Retired Persons. (No date) *A portrait of older minorities.*

Anderson, R. E., and Carter, I. (1974) *Human behavior in the social environment.* (2d ed.) Chicago, IL: Aldine.

Atchley, R. C. (1985) *Social forces and aging: An introduction to social gerontology.* (4th ed.) Belmont, CA: Wadsworth.

Berger, R. M. (1984) Realities of gay and lesbian aging. *Social Work,* 29(1):57–62.

Brieland, D., Costin, L. B., and Atherton, C. R. (1985) *Contemporary social work.* (3d ed.) New York: McGraw-Hill.

Brody, E. M. (1977) *Long-term care of older people: A practical guide.* New York: Human Services Press.

Burghardt, S. (1983) *Organizing for community action.* Beverly Hills, CA: Sage.

Butler, R. N. (1963) The life review: An interpretation of reminiscence in the aged. *Psychiatry* 26:65–76.

Butler, R. N., and Lewis, M. E. (1982) *Aging and mental health.* St. Louis, MO: C. V. Mosby.

Compton, B., and Galaway, B. (1984) *Social work processes.* Chicago, IL: Dorsey.

Cox, F. M., Erlich, J. L., Rothman, J., and Tropman, J. E. (eds.). (1984) *Tactics and techniques of community practice.* Itasca, IL: Peacock.

De Spelder, L. A., and Strickland, A. L. (1987) *The last dance.* (2d ed.) Palo Alto, CA: Mayfield.

Diagnostic and Statistical Manual of Mental Disorders. (3d ed.—Revised) (1988) Washington, DC: American Psychiatric Association.

Ecklein, J. (1984) *Community organizers.* New York: Wiley.

Filley, A. (1975) *Interpersonal conflict resolution.* Glenview, IL: Scott, Foresman.

Garvin, C. D. (1981) *Contemporary group work.* Englewood Cliffs, NJ: Prentice-Hall.

Gavzer, B. (1987, October 13) How secure is your social security? *Parade,* pp. 4–6.

Giordano, N. V. and Giordano, J. A. (1984) Elder abuse: A review of the literature. *Social Work,* 29:232–236.

Gross, B. (1966) The state of the nation: Social systems accounting. In Bauer, Raymond A. (ed.), *Social indicators.* Cambridge, MA: MIT Press.

Harris, L. and associates. (1981) *Aging in the eighties: America in transition.* Washington, DC: National Council on the Aging.

Kane, R. A., and Kane, R. L. (1981) *Assessing the elderly.* Lexington, MA: Lexington Books.

Larson, R. (1978) Thirty years of research on the subjective well-being of older Americans. *Journal of Gerontology, 33:*109–125.

Lawton, M. P., and Nahemow, L. (1973) Ecology and the aging process. In Eisdorfer, C., and Lawton, M. P. (eds.), *Psychology of aging and adult development.* Washington, DC: American Psychological Association.

Lawton, M. P., and Simon, B. (1968) The ecology of social relationships in housing for the elderly. *Gerontologist, 8:*108–115.

Levin, L., and Levin, W. C. (1980) *Ageism: Prejudice and discrimination against the elderly.* Belmont, CA: Wadsworth.

Maslow, A. H. (1954) *Motivation and personality.* New York: Harper.

Monk, A. (1981) Social work with the aged: Principles of practice. *Social Work, 26:*61–63.

Neugarten, B. L. (1981) Personality change in late life: A developmental perspective. In Kart, C. S., and Marand, B. B. (eds.), *Aging in America: Readings in social gerontology.* Sherman Oaks, CA: Alfred.

Peterson, P. G. (1983, March) Can social security be saved? *Reader's Digest,* pp. 49–54.

Reid, W. J. (1978) *The task-centered system.* New York: Columbia University Press.

Roberts, R. W., and Northen, H. (eds.). (1976) *Theories of social work with groups.* New York: Columbia University Press.

Rose, A. M. (1965) The subculture of the aging: A framework for research in social gerontology. In Rose, A. M., and Peterson, W. A. (eds.), *Older people and their social worlds.* Philadelphia, PA: F. A. Davis.

Rubin, A., and Johnson, P. (1982) Practitioner orientations toward the chronically disabled. *Administration in Mental Health, 10:*3–12.

Schorr, Alvin. (1980) . . . *Thy father and thy mother . . . a second look at familial responsibility and family policy.* Washington, DC: Department of Health and Human Services.

Schulz, J. H. (1985) *The economics of aging.* Belmont, CA: Wadsworth.

Skellie, F. A., and Coan, R. E. (1980) Community-based long-term care and mortality: Preliminary findings of Georgia's alternative health services project. *Gerontologist, 20:*372–379.

Social security in review. (1988) *Social Security Bulletin, 51*(1):2–3.

Sontag, S. (1972) The double standard of aging. *Saturday Review, 55:*29–38.

Stone, L. J., and Church, J. (1973) *Childhood and adolescence.* New York: Random House.

Stuart, P., and Rathbone-McCuan, E. (1988) Indian elderly in the United States. In Rathbone-McCuan, E., and Havens, B. (eds.), *North American elders: Canadian and U.S. comparison.* Westport, CT: Greenwood.

Taber, M. A., Anderson, S., and Rogers, C. J. (1980) Implementing community care in Illinois: Issues of cost and targeting in a statewide program. *Gerontologist, 20*:380–387.

U.S. Bureau of the Census. (1986) *Statistical abstract of the United States: 1987.* (107th ed.) Washington, DC: U.S. Government Printing Office.

U.S. Senate Special Committee on Aging. (1984) *Aging America.* Washington, DC: Department of Health and Human Services.

U.S. Senate Special Committee on Aging. (1985) *Aging in America: Trends and projections.* Washington, DC: Department of Health and Human Services.

World Health Organizations. (1946) Constitution of the world health organization. *Public Health Report, 61*:1268–1277.

Wood, J. B., and Estes, C. L. (1988) "Medicalization" of community services for the elderly. *Health and Social Work, 13*(1):35–42.

Ycas, M. A., and Grad, S. (1987) Income of retirement-aged persons in the United States. *Social Security Bulletin, 50*(7):5–14.

Index